NUDIST CAMP FOLLIES

VOLUME II

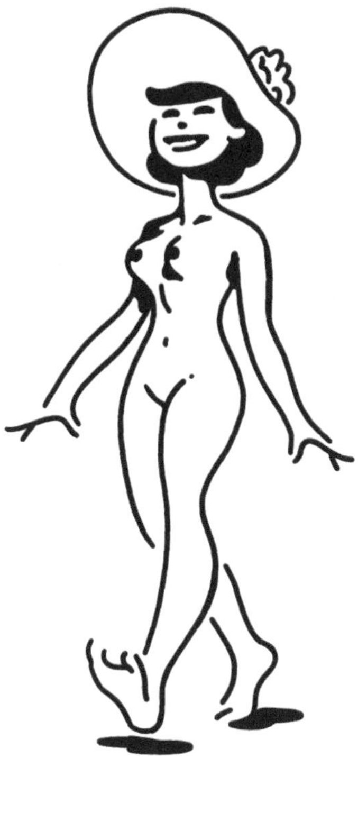

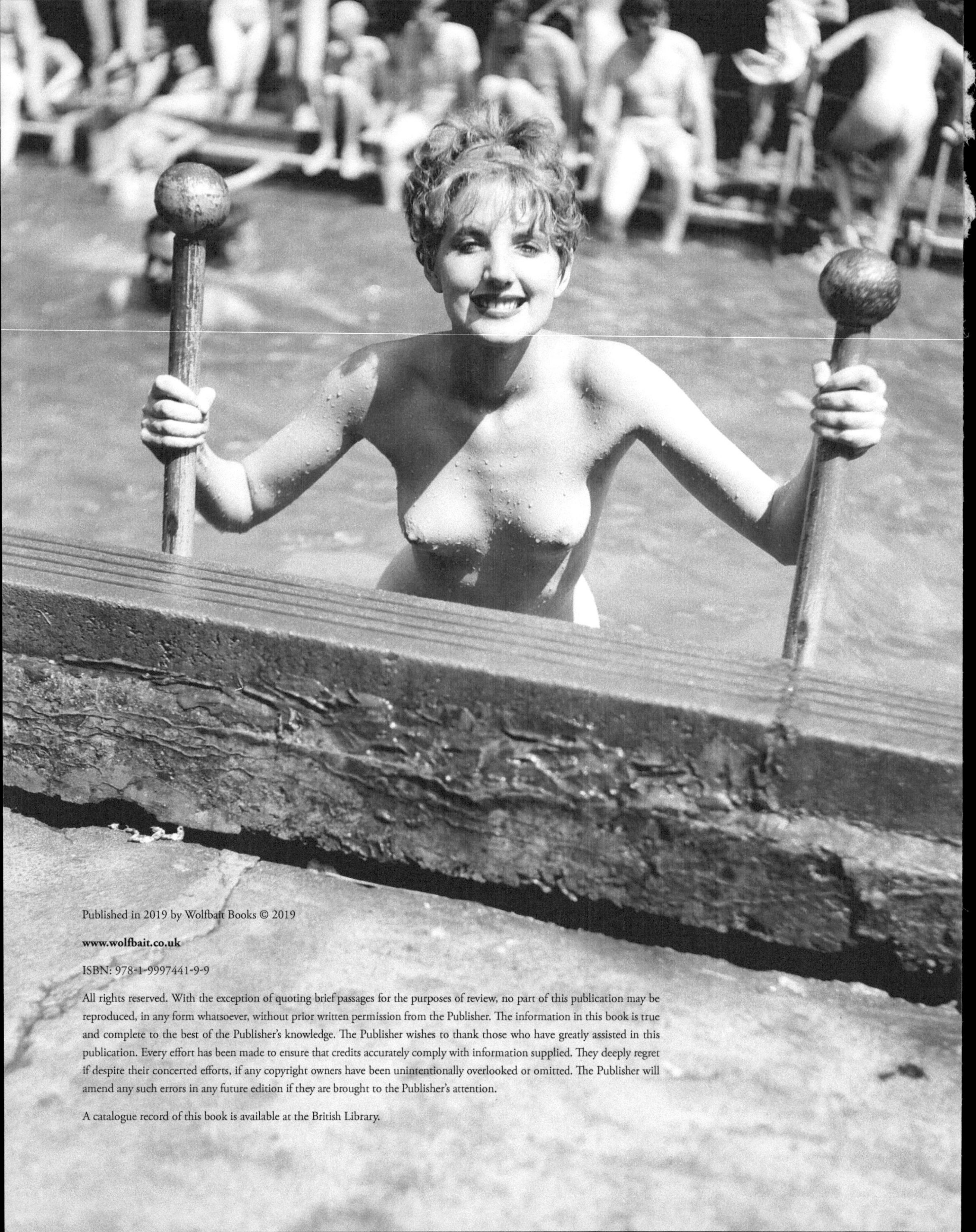

Published in 2019 by Wolfbait Books © 2019

www.wolfbait.co.uk

ISBN: 978-1-9997441-9-9

A catalogue record of this book is available at the British Library.

NUDIST CAMP FOLLIES

VOLUME II

By Yahya El-Droubie
Photography by Stephen Glass
Illustrations by Colin Gordon

WOLFBAIT
UNDER THE COUNTER CULTURE

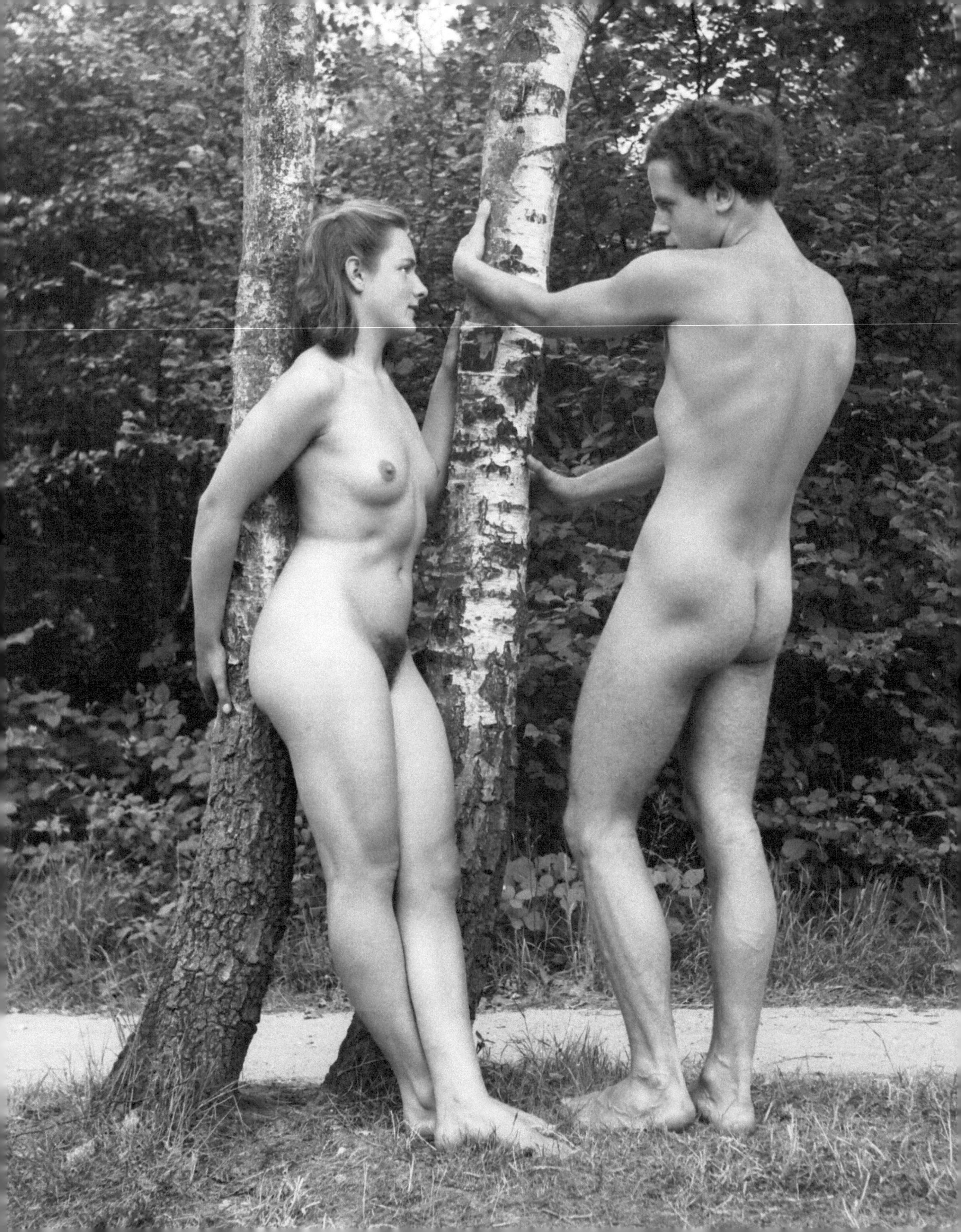

Introduction

THE PHOTOGRAPHER STEPHEN GLASS is something of an enigma. He was sufficiently well-known during the 1950s for his name to be prominently displayed on magazine covers to help sell them, but very little was written about him or his work at that time. The opposite is true of his elder brother, Zoltán, who was also a photographer. Known to his friends as "Zolly", Zoltán was featured and interviewed in numerous magazines on both sides of the Atlantic.

Zoltán Glass was born in Budapest, Hungary, on April 26, 1903. He began his career as a cartoonist and retoucher for a local newspaper, but in 1925 he moved to Berlin, where he was employed as the picture editor of an evening newspaper; he then moved on to the *Berliner Tagblatt* as a photojournalist. Zoltán prospered and was soon able to develop a thriving freelance business as a commercial photographer and journalist. He established Reclaphot, a photographic agency that specialised in advertising work, and Autophot, a company dedicated exclusively to automobile photography. A keen motor sport enthusiast and amateur racer, Zoltán covered Germany's biggest races at the Nürburgring and Avus circuits. His famous photographs are of the Mercedes-Benz Silver Arrows team, which dominated Grand Prix racing in the mid-1930s.

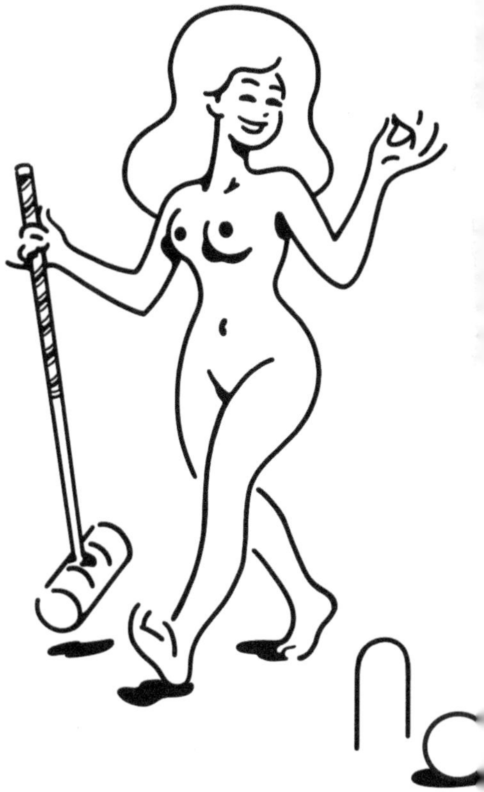

With the rise of Hitler, business became increasingly difficult in Germany, and Zoltán fled to London. As an enemy alien at the outbreak of World War II, he was not permitted to pursue his profession and faced the threat of internment, so he voluntarily handed over his camera equipment to the British authorities.

After the war, Zoltán eked out a living taking publicity stills for clients in the film and theatre worlds. His career took a big step up when fellow Hungarian Arpad Elfer, Creative Director of Colman, Prentis & Varley, one of the most prestigious London ad agencies, started giving him work. By the mid-1950s, he was one of the most successful fashion and advertising photographers in the capital, with a studio at 183 Kings Road, Chelsea, and later another at 41 Paradise Walk, SW3.

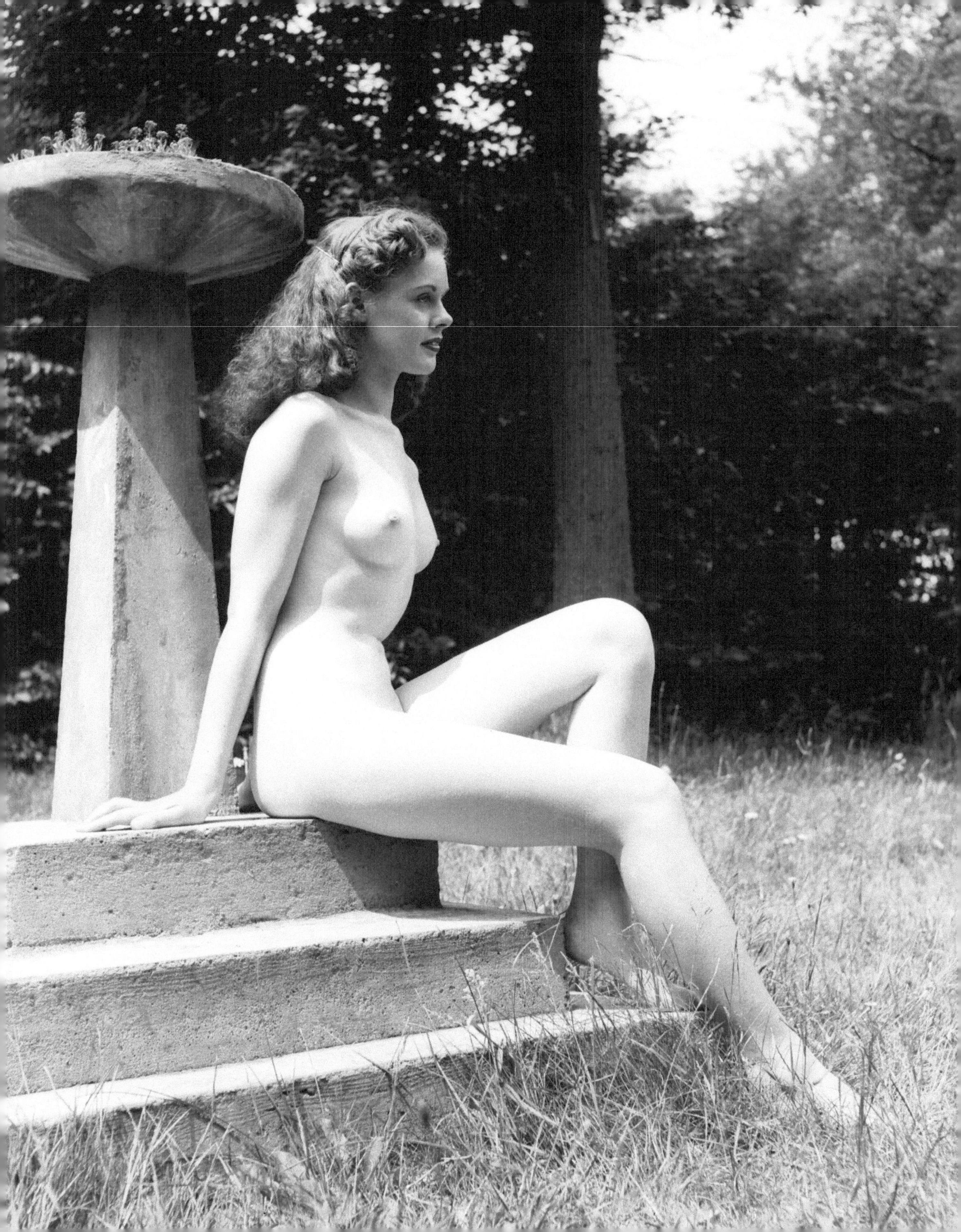

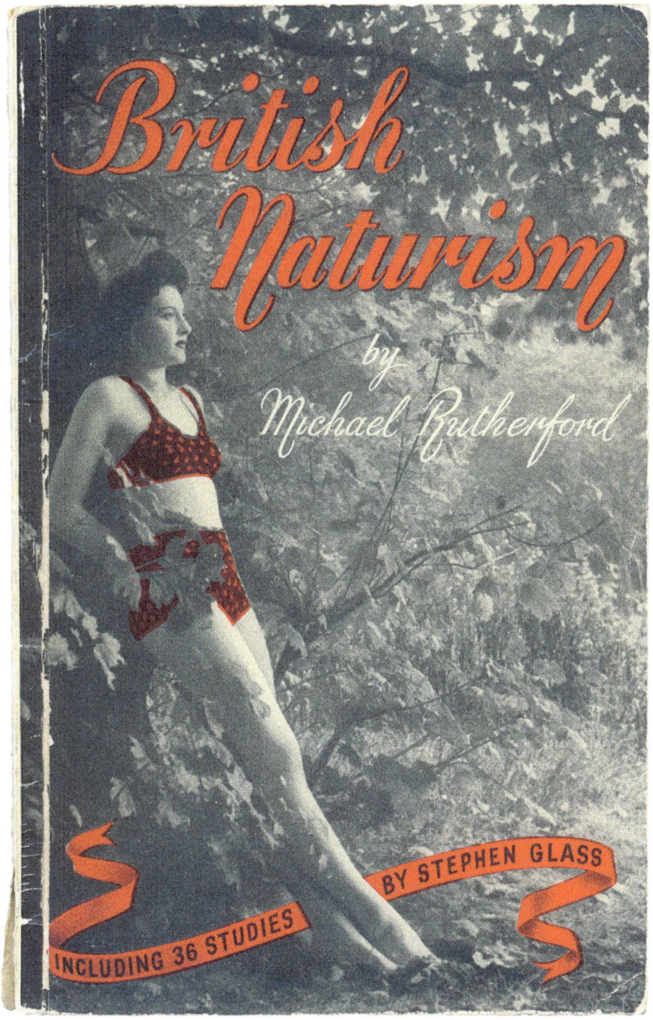

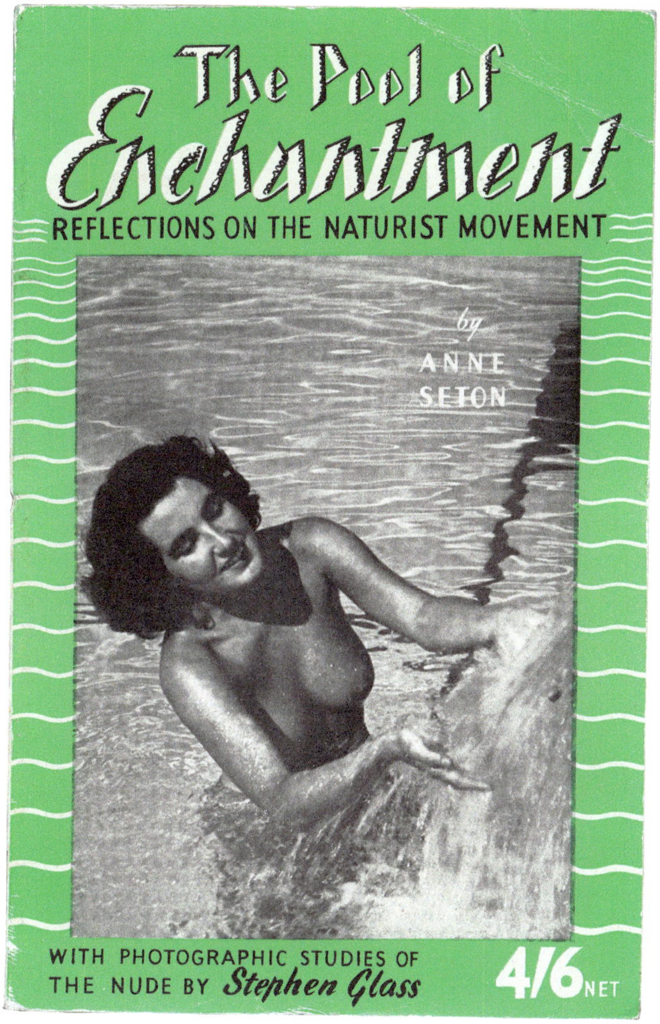

One of his clients was Odhams Press, who published *Lilliput*, a pocket-sized gentleman's magazine that featured an assortment of titillating articles and risqué humour, together with adventurous photographic essays from such well-known talents as Bill Brandt and Brassai.

Zoltán's brother, Stephen, who also fled Europe during World War II, carved out a name for himself taking pictures for such publications as *The Naturist* and *Health and Efficiency.* The well-known model Pamela Green (1929–2010) posed for him several times at the infamous nudist camp Spielplatz in Bricket Wood, Hertfordshire, and at his tiny first-floor studio in Old Church Street, just off the Kings Road in Chelsea. *"In those days, when Stephen photographed me, I still had*

Above left: *British Naturism* by Michael Rutherford, published by The Naturist Ltd., 1946.

Above right: *The Pool of Enchantment: Reflections on the Naturist Movement* by Anne Seton, published by The Naturist Ltd, 1950.

Far left: Cover image of *Health and Efficiency*, January 1951.

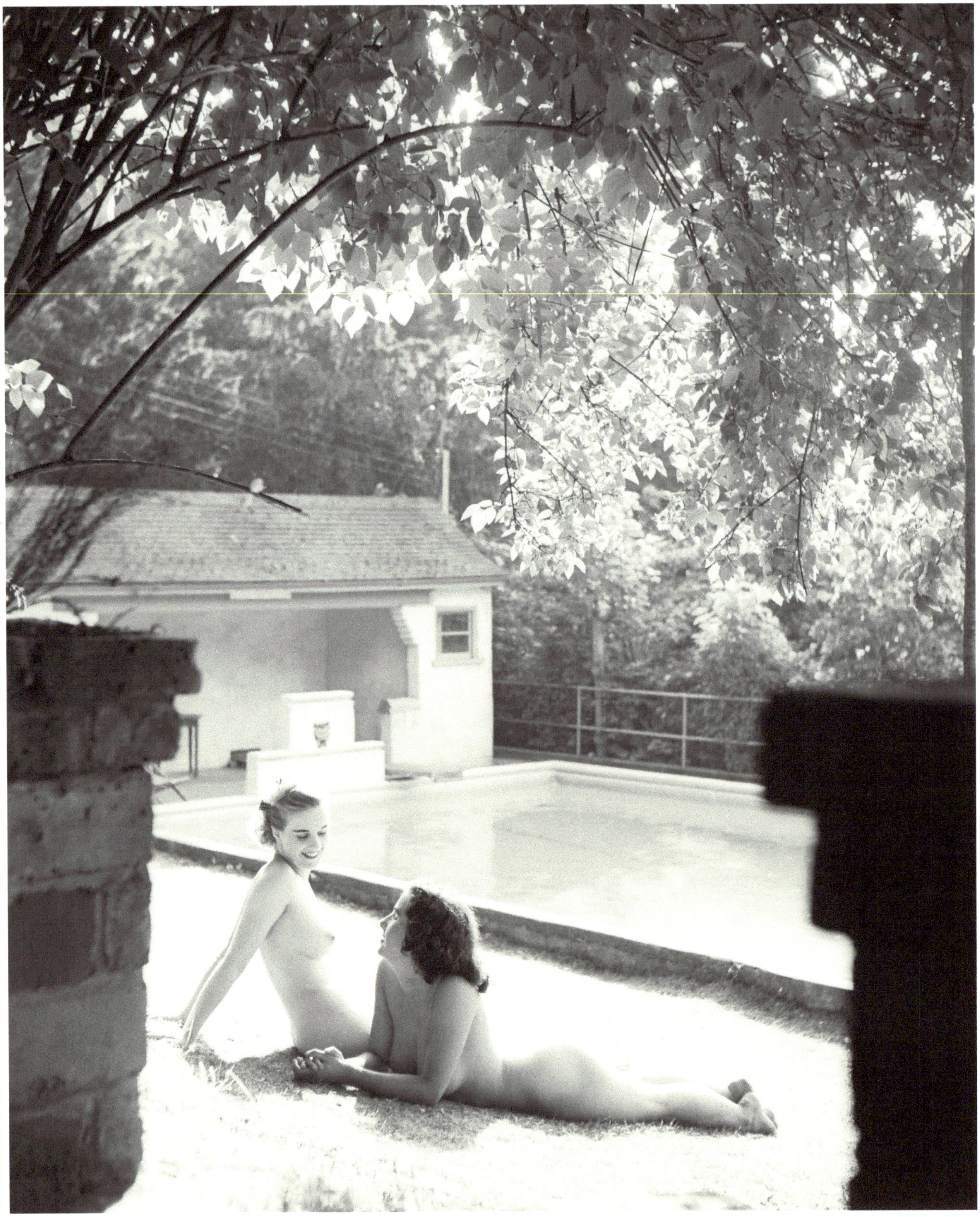

dark hair. He liked his props, especially stuffed animals," she said. Pamela's agent, Pearl Beresford, sent her along to Zoltán, whose studio on the Kings Road was enormous by comparison. Unlike Stephen, Zoltán was brisk and businesslike.

Iseult, the daughter of Spielplatz co-founders Charles and Dorothy Macaskie, remembers Stephen. *"He would often ask me to pose for him,"* she said. *"I quite enjoyed having my photo taken, but when I asked to be paid, he stopped using me. A bit of pocket money back then would have been nice."*

As well as magazines, Stephen's work graced a series of small books published by The Naturist Ltd., such as *Sussex Maidens* (1949), *The Pool of Enchantment* (1950) and *Nudist Life in Spielplatz* (1956). He also photographed the popular model June Palmer (1940–2004). The photos in this book are from his uncensored negatives.

Until the end of the 1960s, it was considered obscene to show pubic hair or genitalia in British publications. To ensure an image of a naked young lady would not incur the wrath of the censor, the model would shave down below and the photograph would then be retouched by hand to erase anything problematic.

By 1964, Zoltán Glass had made enough money to sell his Chelsea studios to a consortium of British photographers. He then moved to a villa in Roquebrune on the French Riviera, with his common-law wife Pat, a former cabaret dancer. He offered his collection of pin-up photography to glamour photographer Harrison Marks who, strangely, turned it down. Zoltán died in France on February 24, 1981, at the age of 78, leaving neither offspring nor a will. His photographs were eventually given to The National Science and Media Museum in Bradford, Yorkshire. Stephen Glass died on 23 April, 1990. His work ended up at auction.

Nudism is not a class movement; among its adherents will be found naval and military officers, doctors, members of the Bar, middle-class businessmen and women, clerks and typists. They are just ordinary people, even if their notions may seem somewhat eccentric to the uninitiated.

— William Welby, *The Naked Truth about Nudism*, 1941.

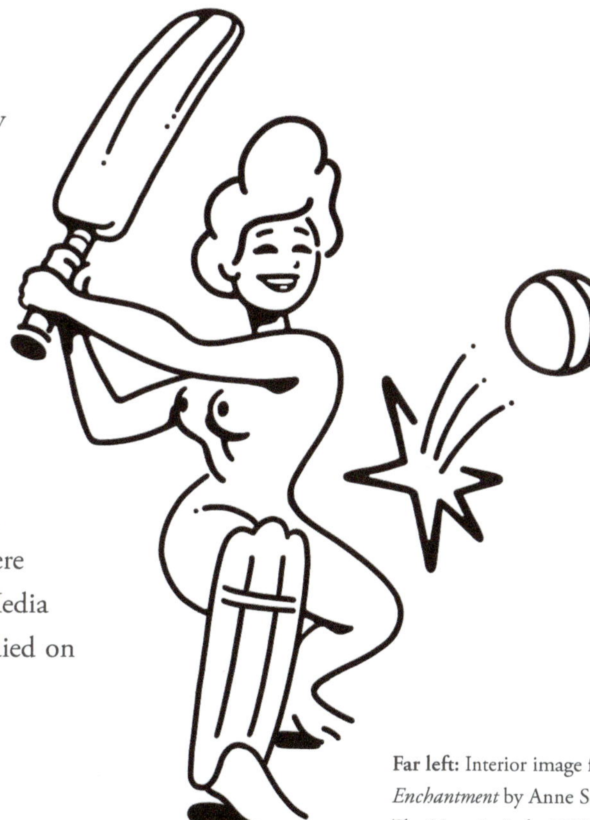

Far left: Interior image from *The Pool of Enchantment* by Anne Seton, published by The Naturist Ltd., 1950.

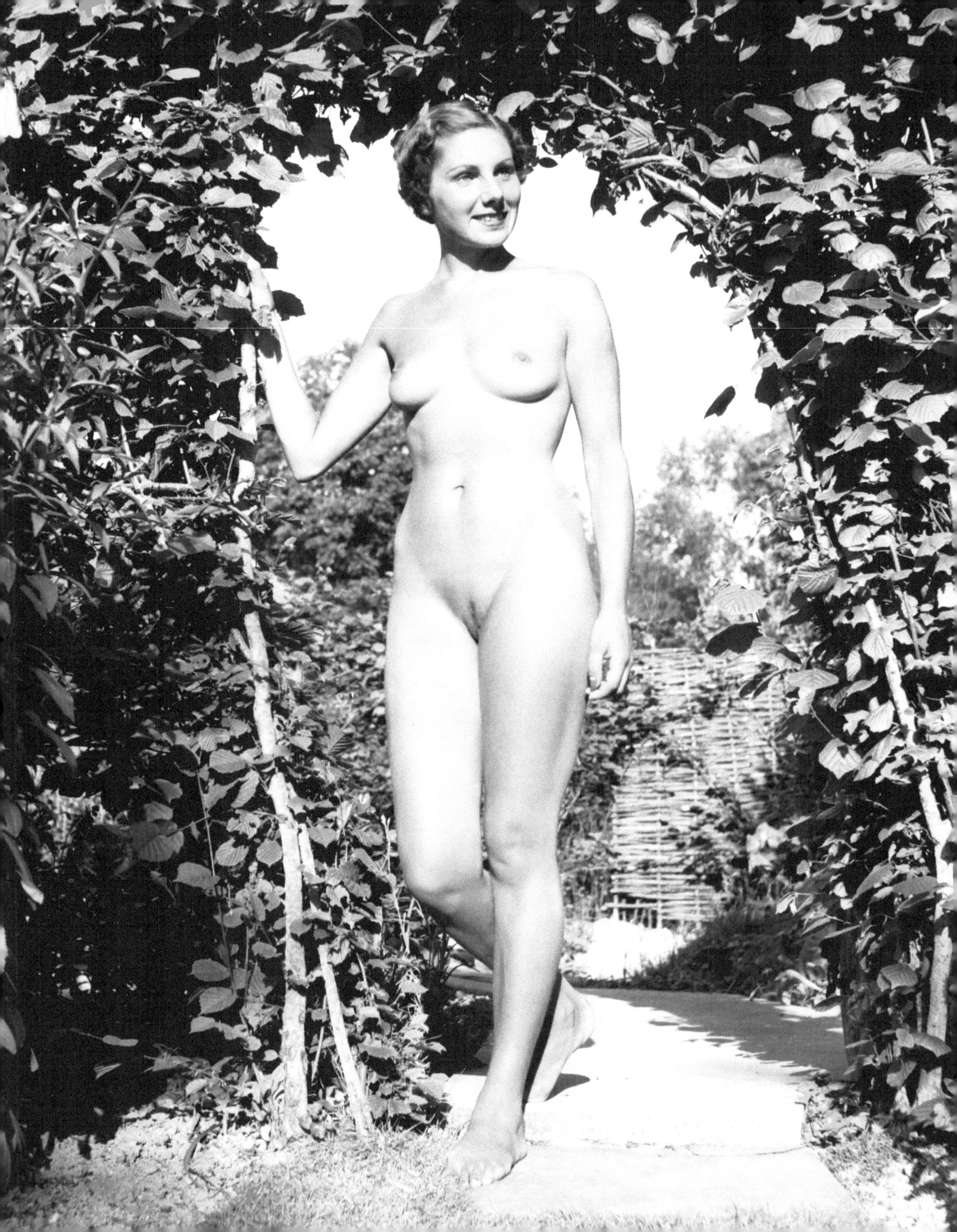

Many of those who posed in naturist resorts for photographers such as Stephen Glass were professional models rather than genuine naturists. One of the handful to buck that trend was Elizabeth Walker, née Elcoate Gilbert, who was routinely described as Naturism's Ambassador. She was a member of Spielplatz and as early as 1950, regularly featured in magazines such as *Health and Efficiency* and *The Naturist*. In 1955 she met former RAF pilot Edward Craven Walker at Spileplatz. Craven Walker found fame and riches as the inventor of the lava lamp, but he was also something of an evangelist for the naturist movement. Not only did he set up his own nudist camp near Ringwood in Hampshire, called the Bournemouth and District Outdoor Club, he directed and produced three films on naturism under the pseudonym Michael Keatering.

Travelling Light (1959) was one of the first naturist films to receive a public release in the UK. It stars Elizabeth Walker – performing in the all-together – who is invited to join some naturists on a trip to the famous nudist colony at Villata in Corsica. There, they meet Yannick, who performs a unique "underwater ballet". At the end of her holiday, Elizabeth returns home naturally refreshed with a newfound enthusiasm and understanding for naturism.

Sunswept (1961) was the next film in the trilogy. In this, Elizabeth, now a committed naturist, goes to her local sun club, where she meets some newlyweds who are about to go on their honeymoon to France. The film turns into a continental travelogue of famous nudist sites, such as the Isle of Levant and the nudist beach on the island of Rab in Yugoslavia. Yannick, from the first film, also makes a guest appearance. As a nudist film made by a real nudist, it was awarded the first-ever Certificate of Approval by the British Federation of Sun Clubs.

Sick of beaches and beach balls, Craven Walker's final film, which also starred Elizabeth, was *Eves on Skis* (1963). Frolicking over sand dunes and messing about in the sea were replaced by skiing, throwing snowballs and building igloos in the Austrian Alps. What's not to like?

By 1964 Elizabeth and Craven Walker had separated. Elizabeth went on to run an aromatherapy massage business, and remained a nudist all her life. Craven Walker lost much of his film archive when a tree fell on the garage in which it was stored while he was at Costa Natura, a naturist resort in Málaga, Spain.

Nudism was a contentious topic in 1950s Britain, and its wholesome underlying ideology was exploited by salacious filmmakers eager to sneak nudity past the British censor and onto cinema screens. The first of many nudist films at British cinemas was *Nudist Paradise* (1958), while the most notorious was probably *Naked As Nature Intended* (1961), by George Harrison Marks. Both included scenes shot at Spielplatz. Even the well-known director Michael Winner dabbled in the genre, with the film *Some Like it Cool* (1961).

Far left: Naturism's Ambassador, Elizabeth Walker, wife of Edward Craven Walker, the inventor of the lava lamp.

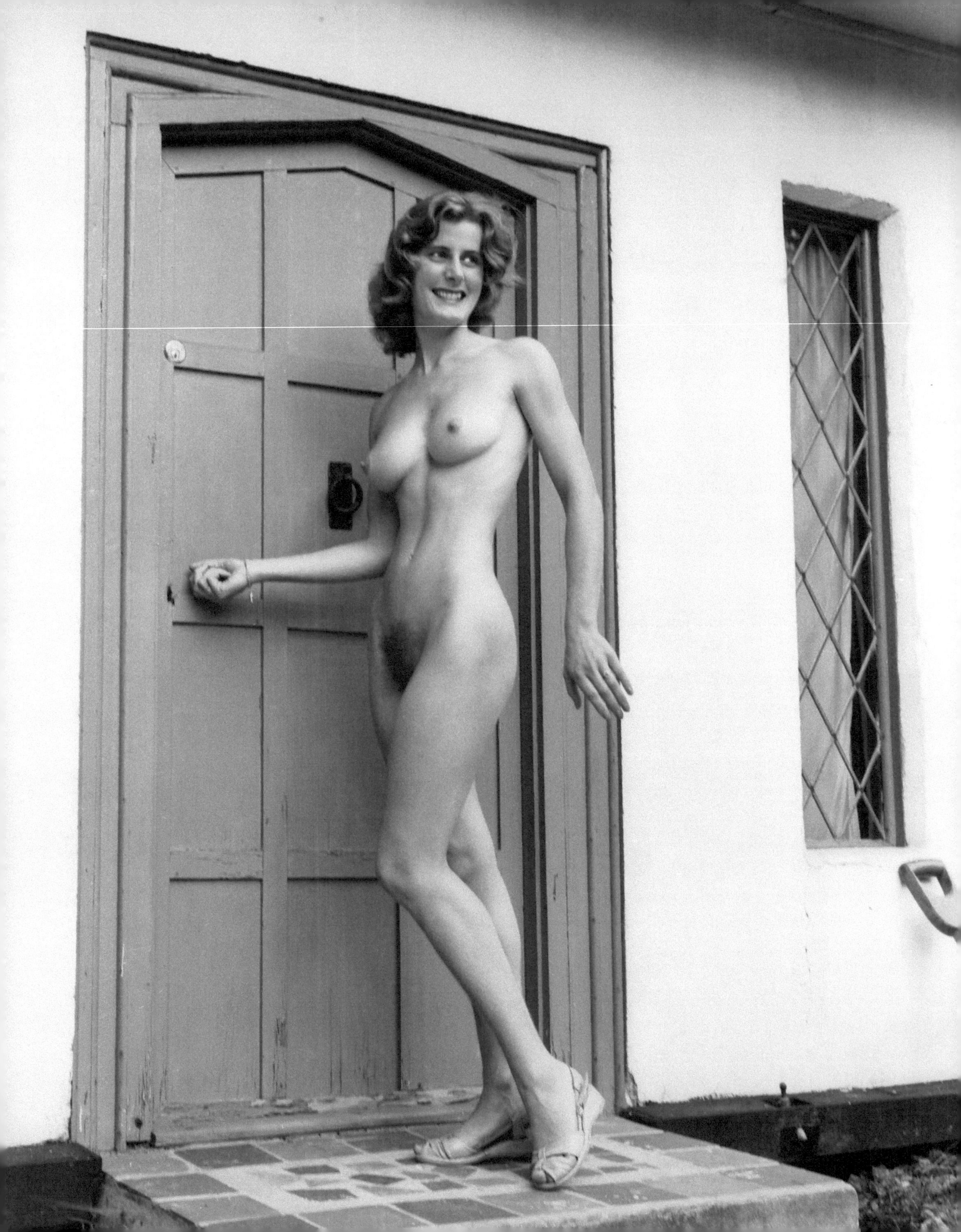

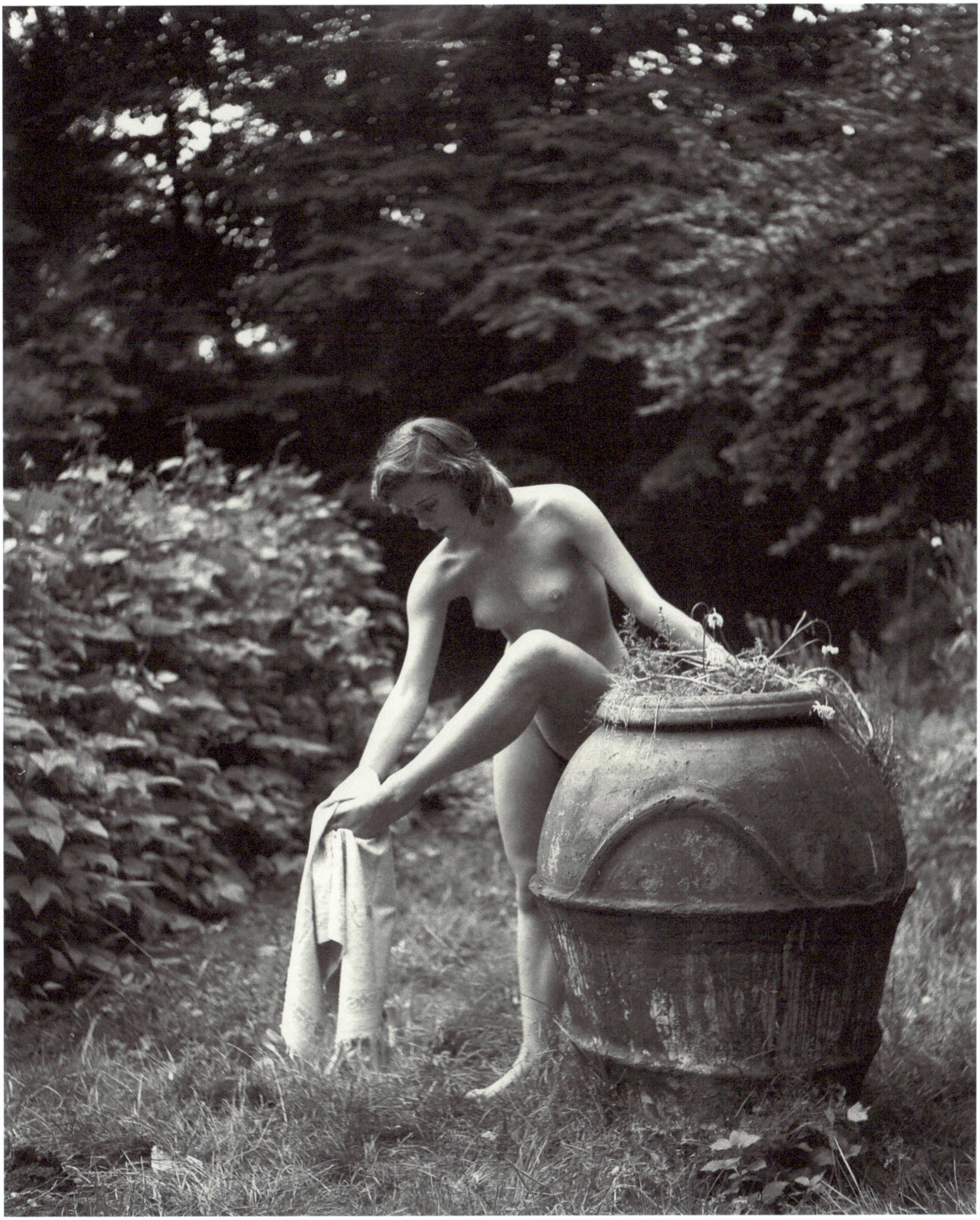

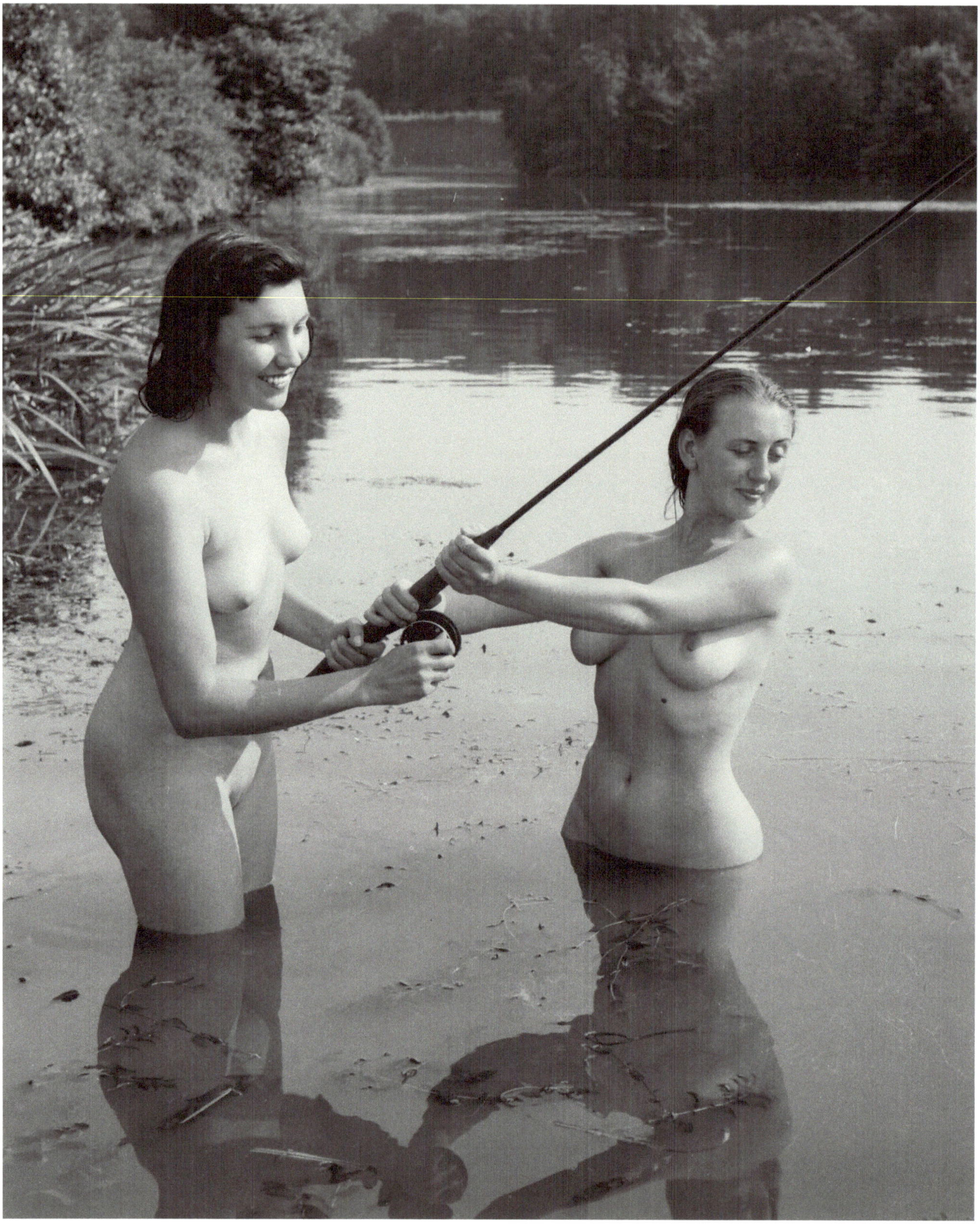

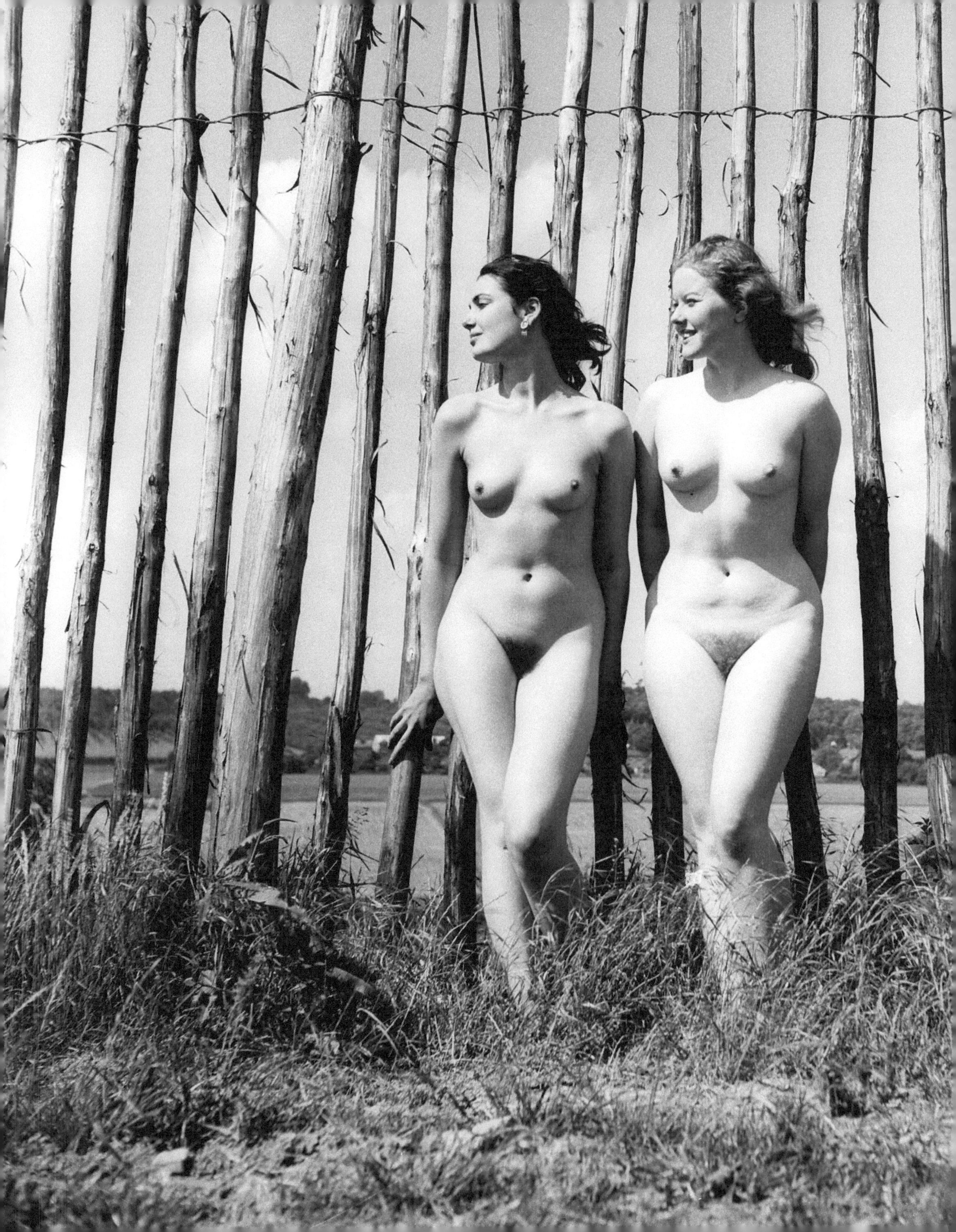

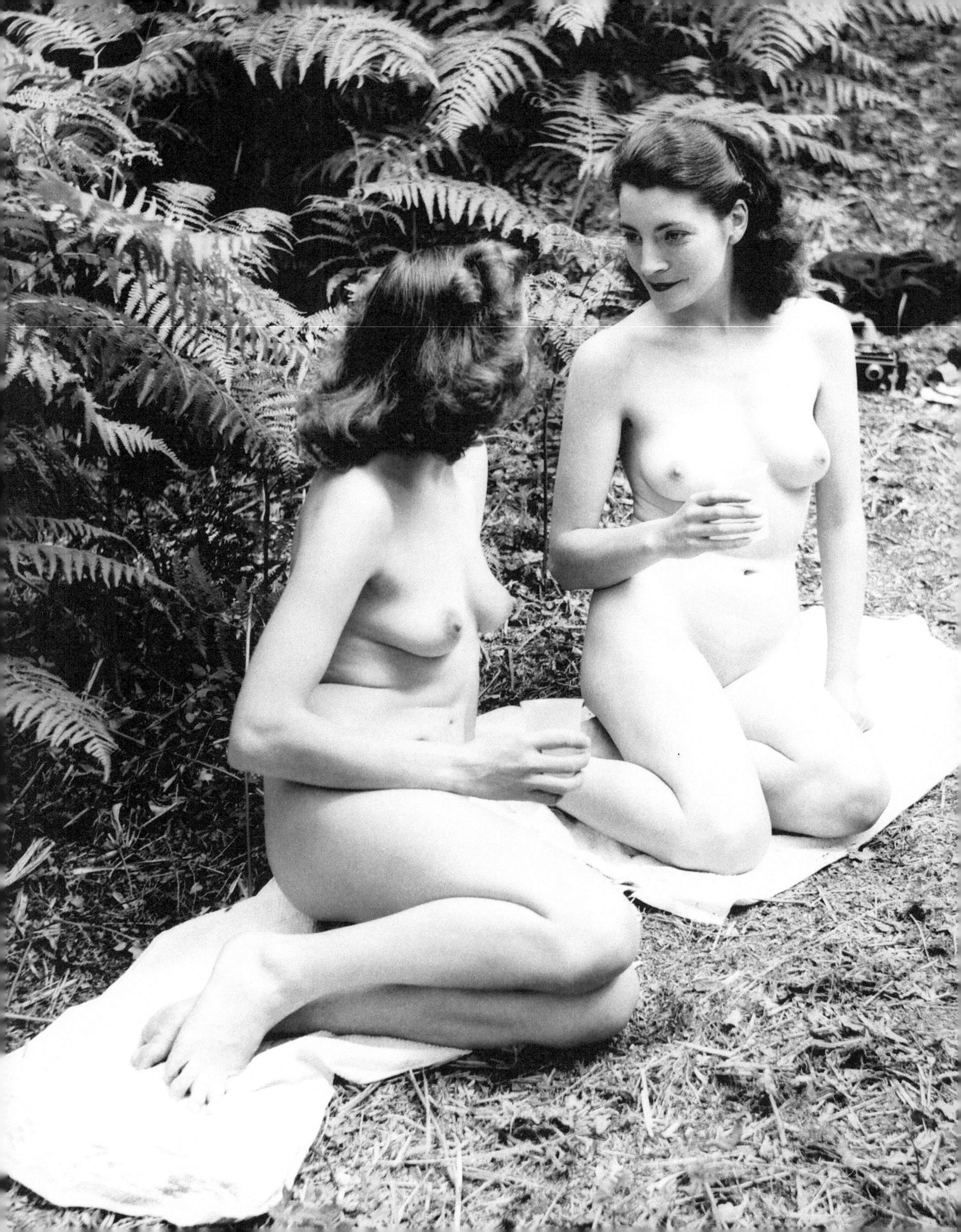

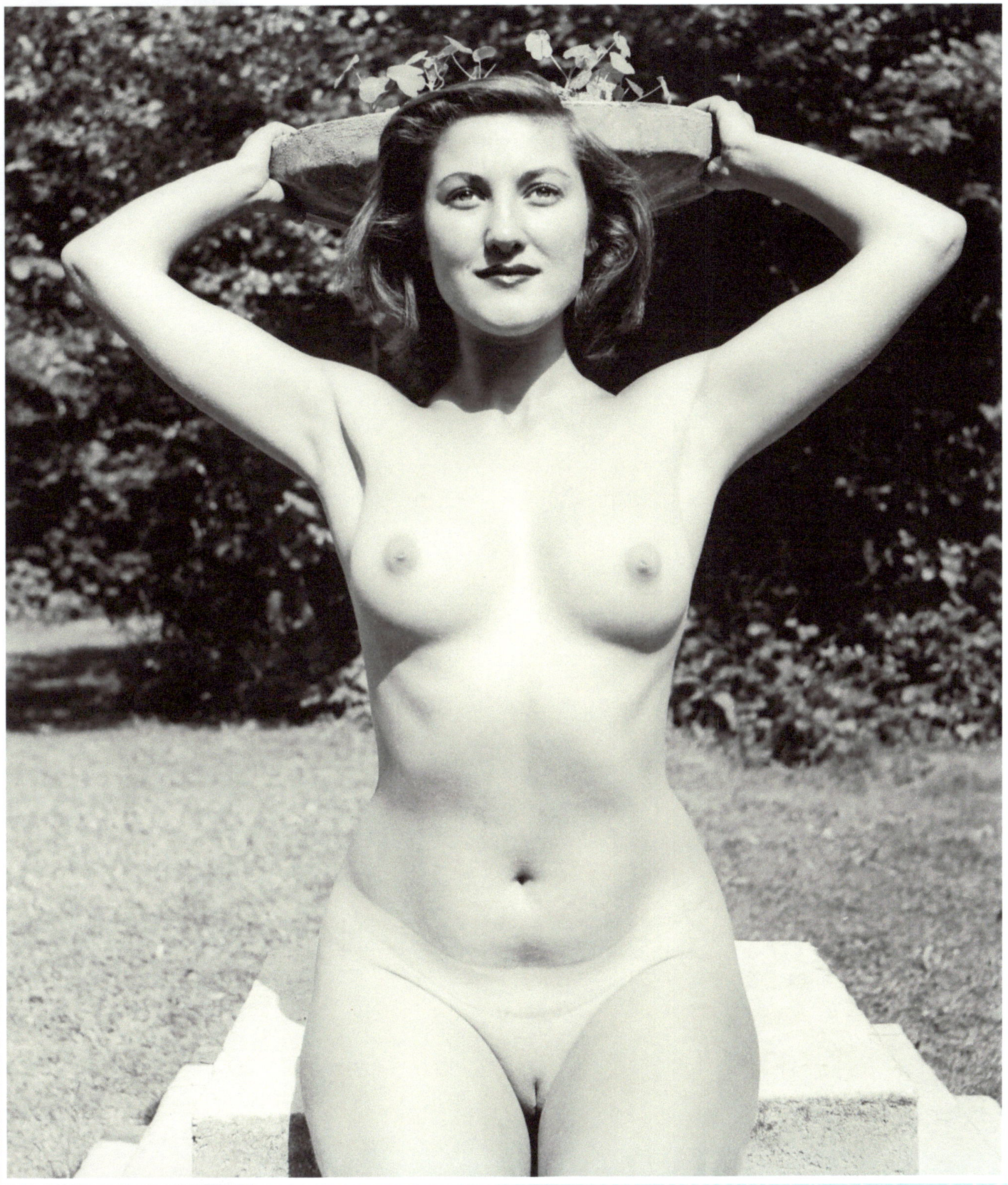

Above: Barbara Thourgood.

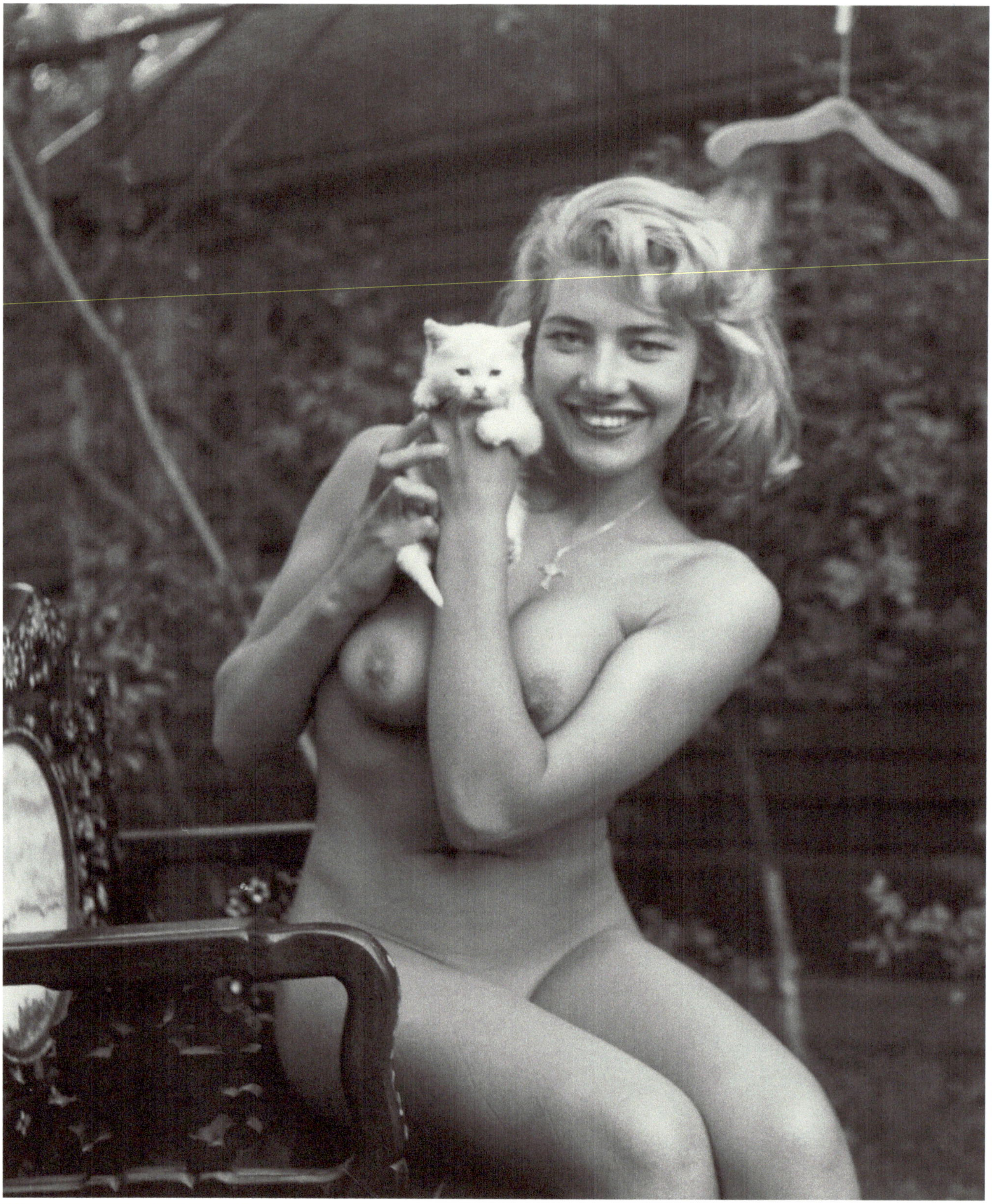

Above: Nancy Roberts.

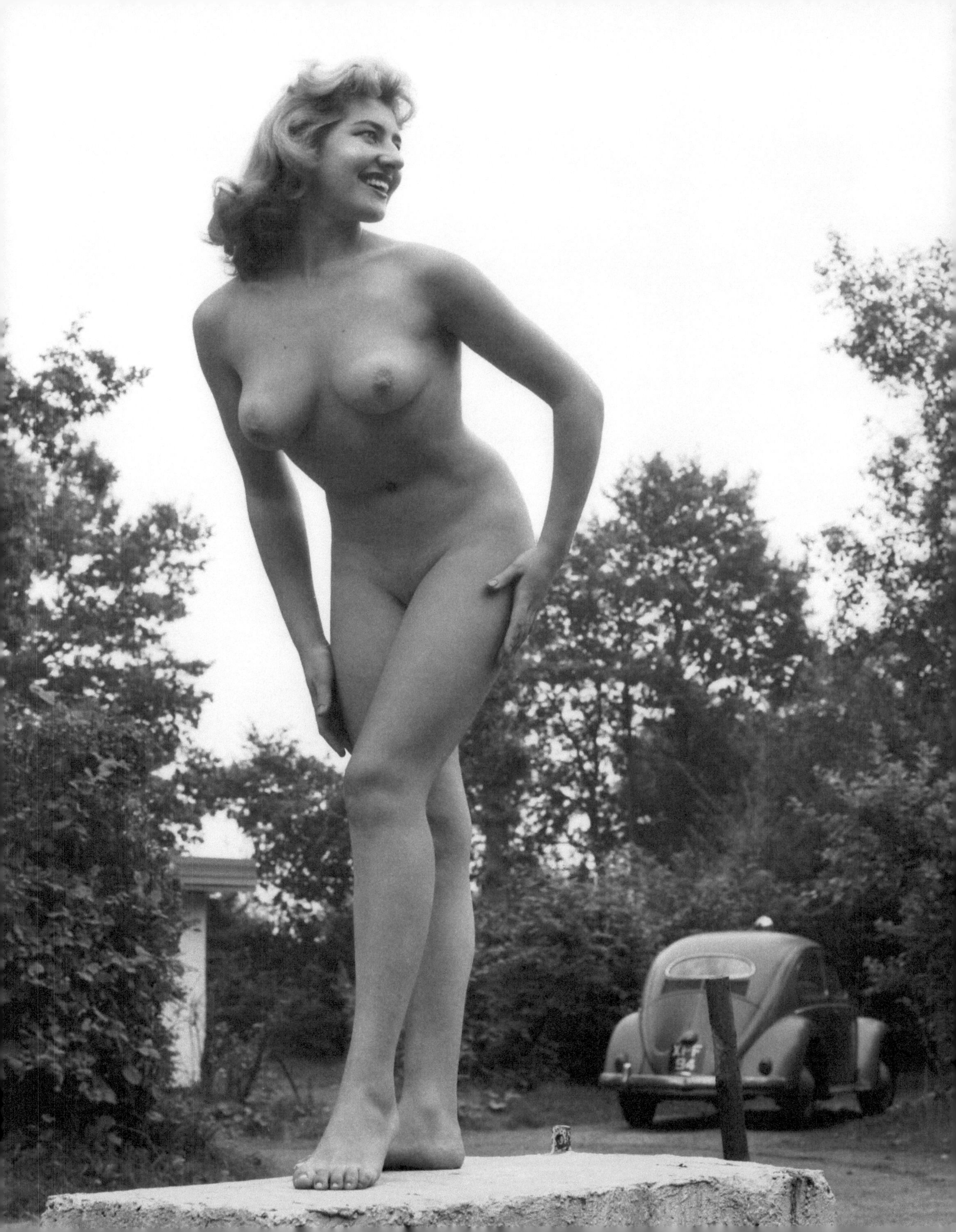

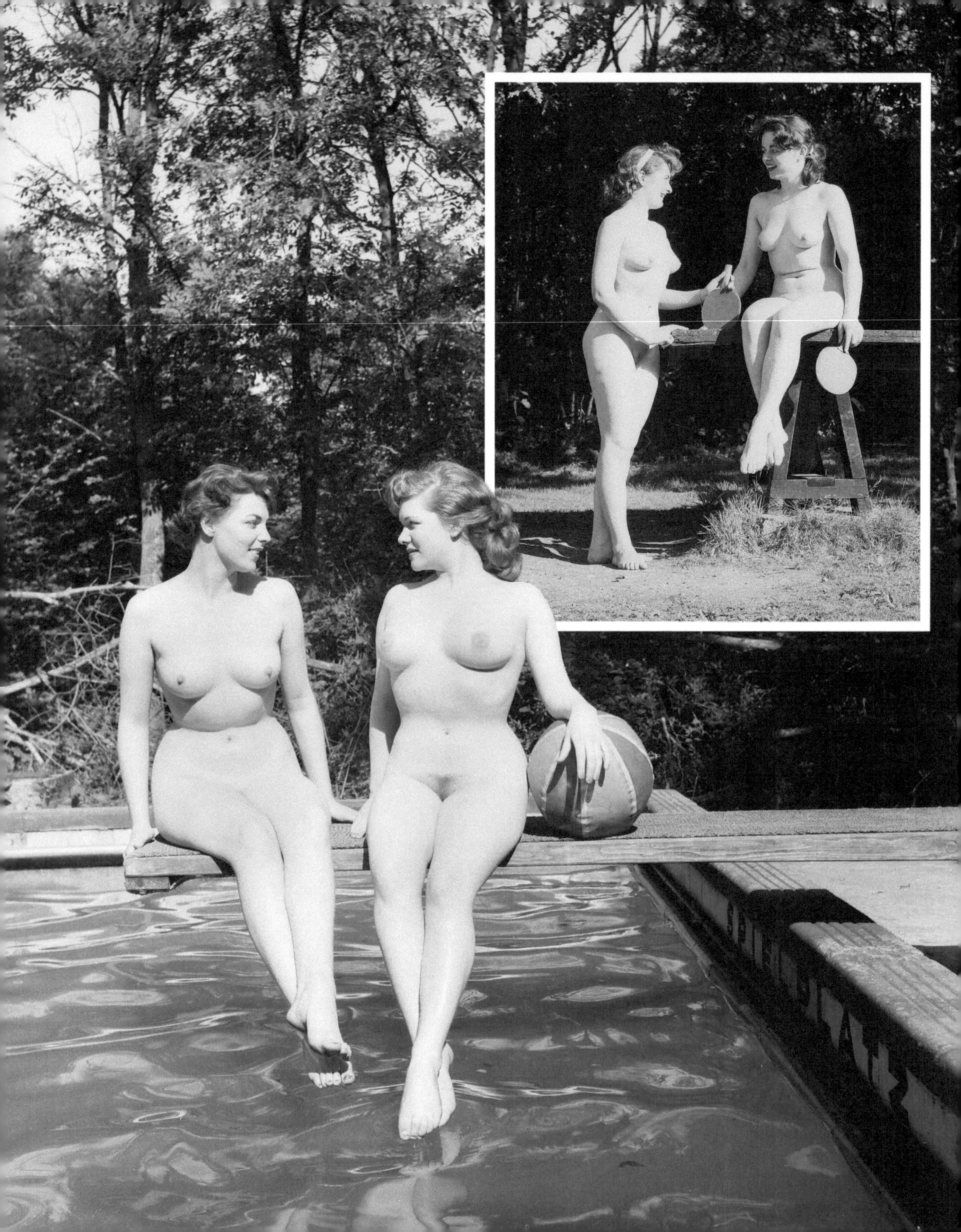

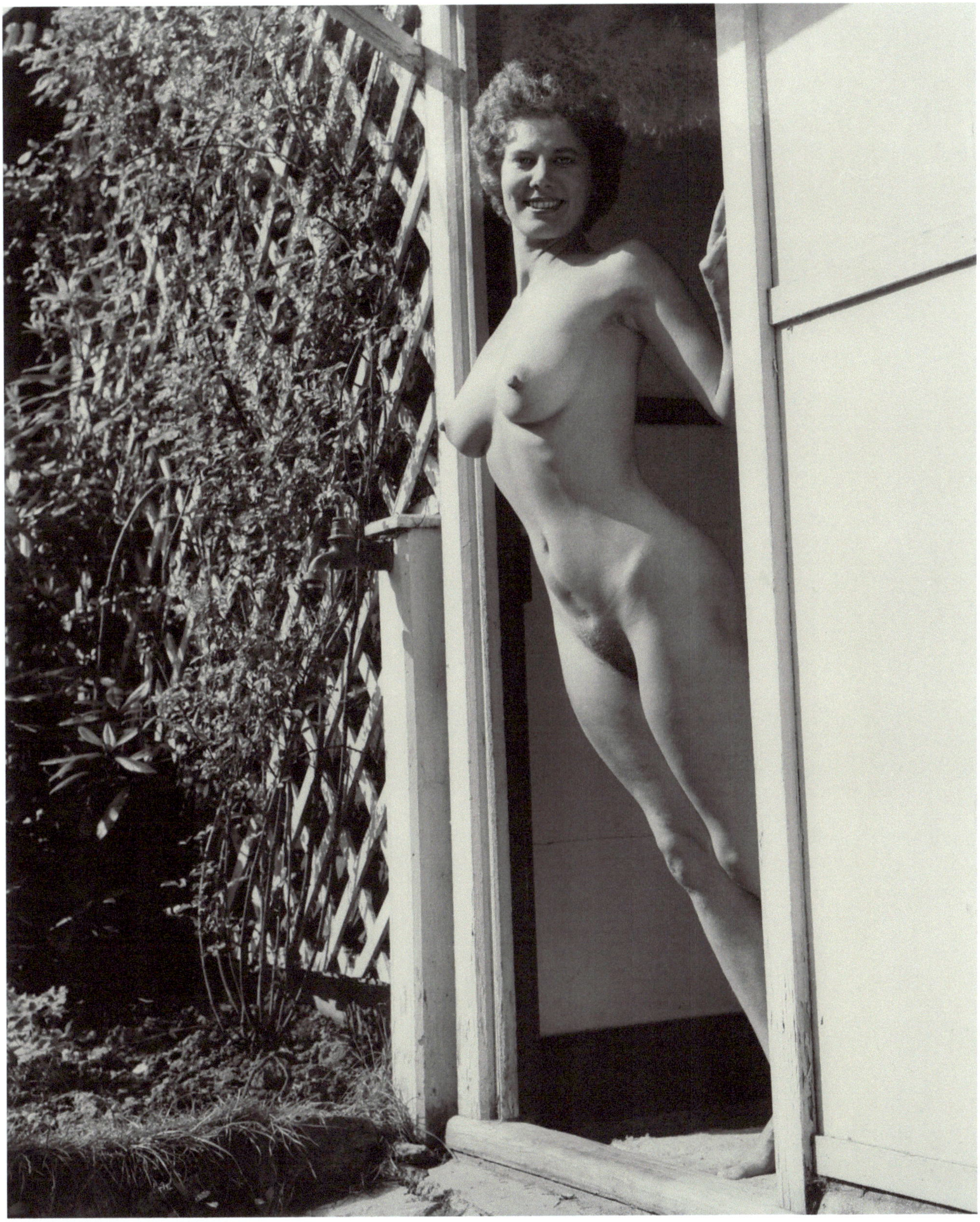

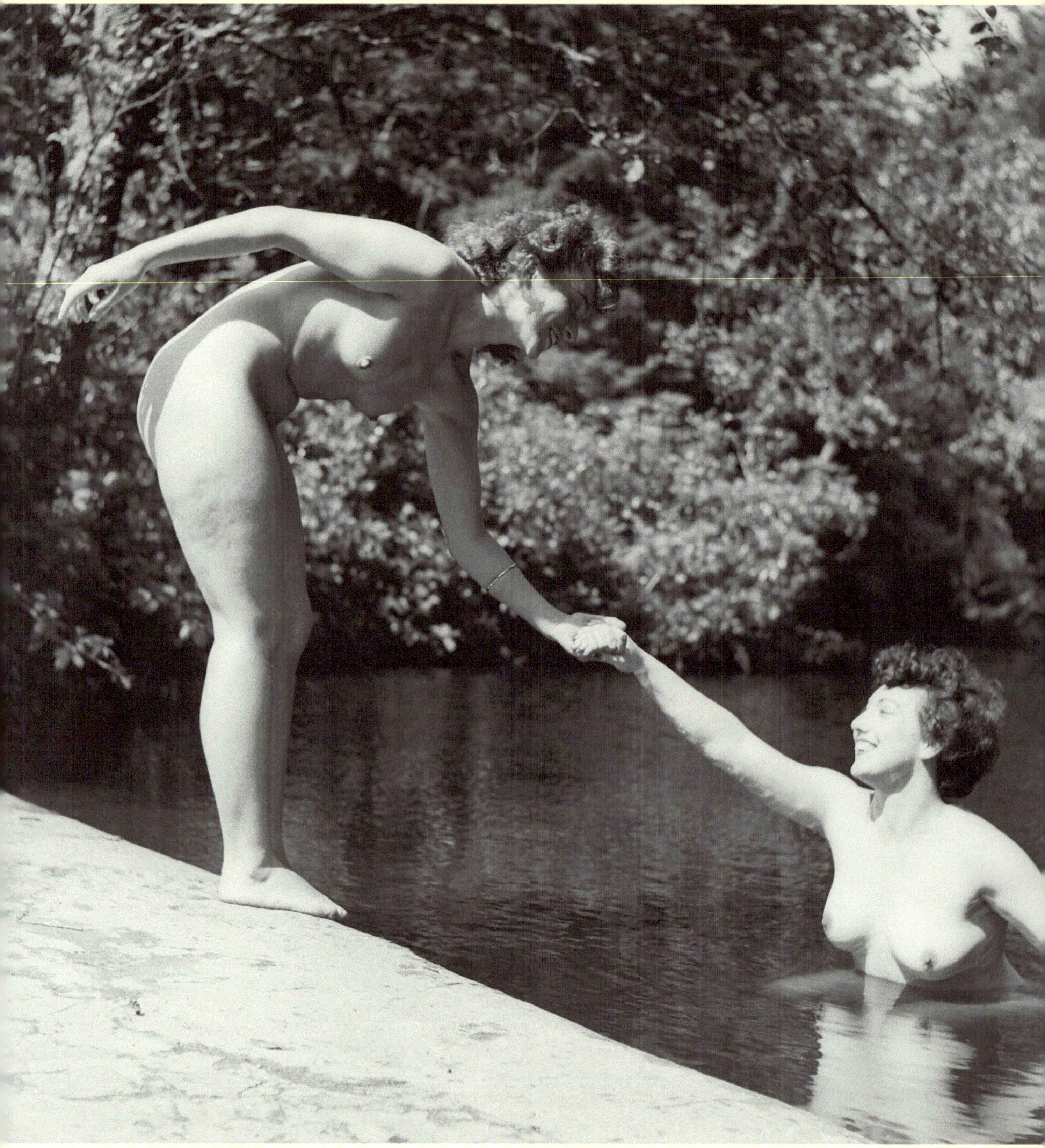

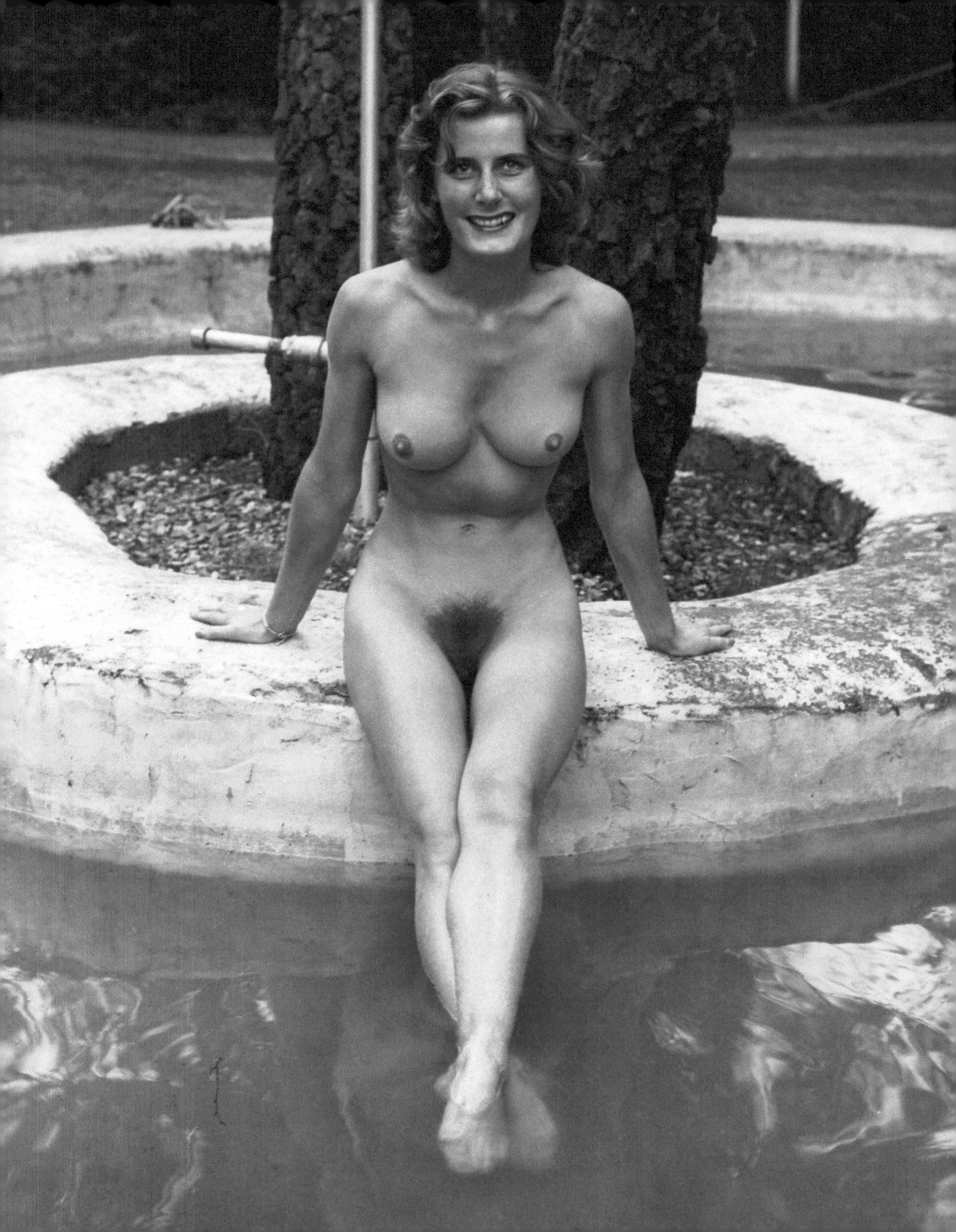

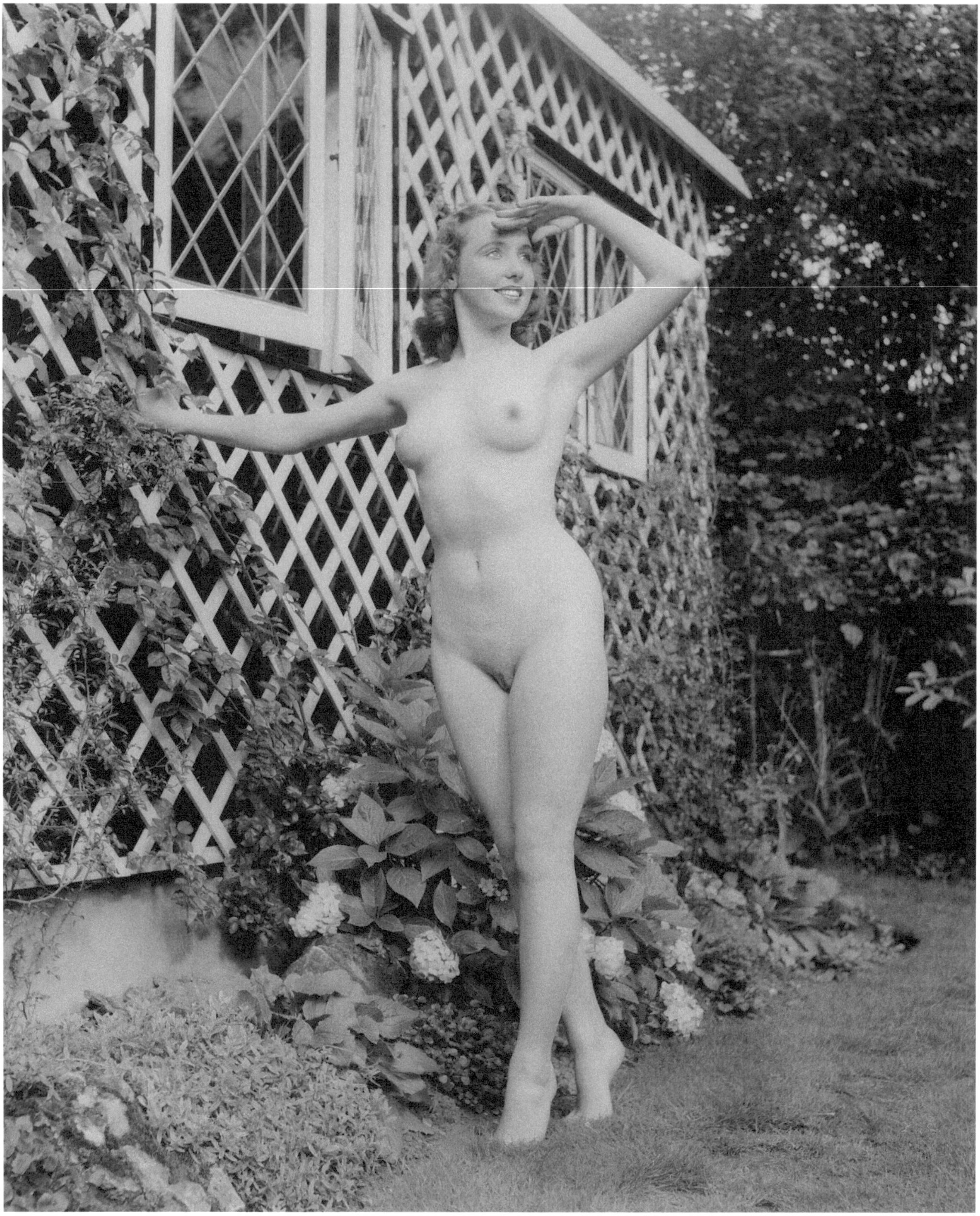

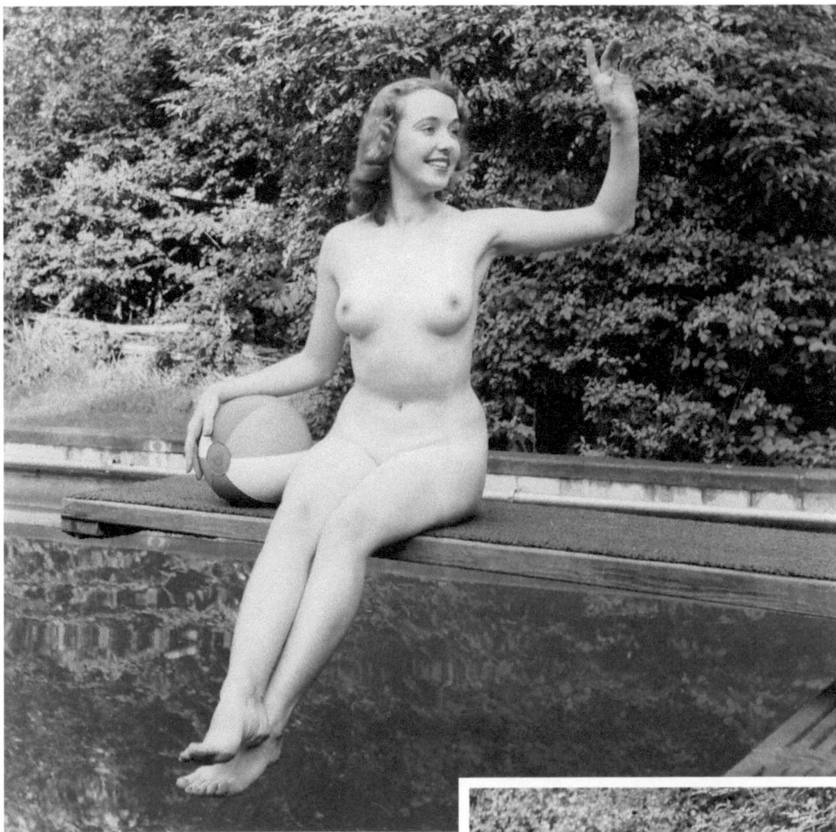

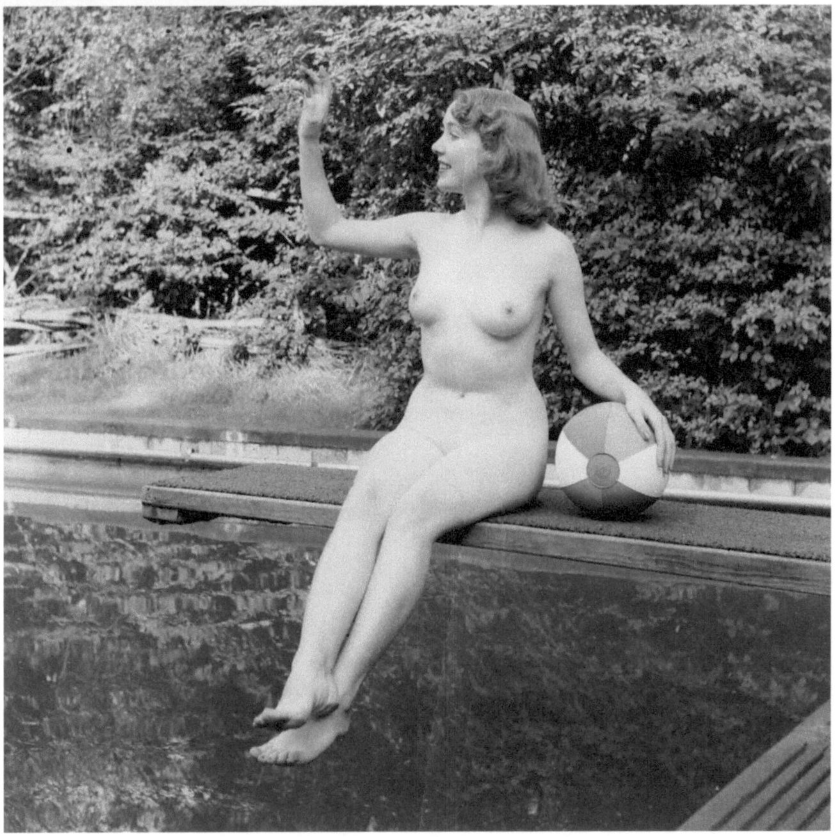

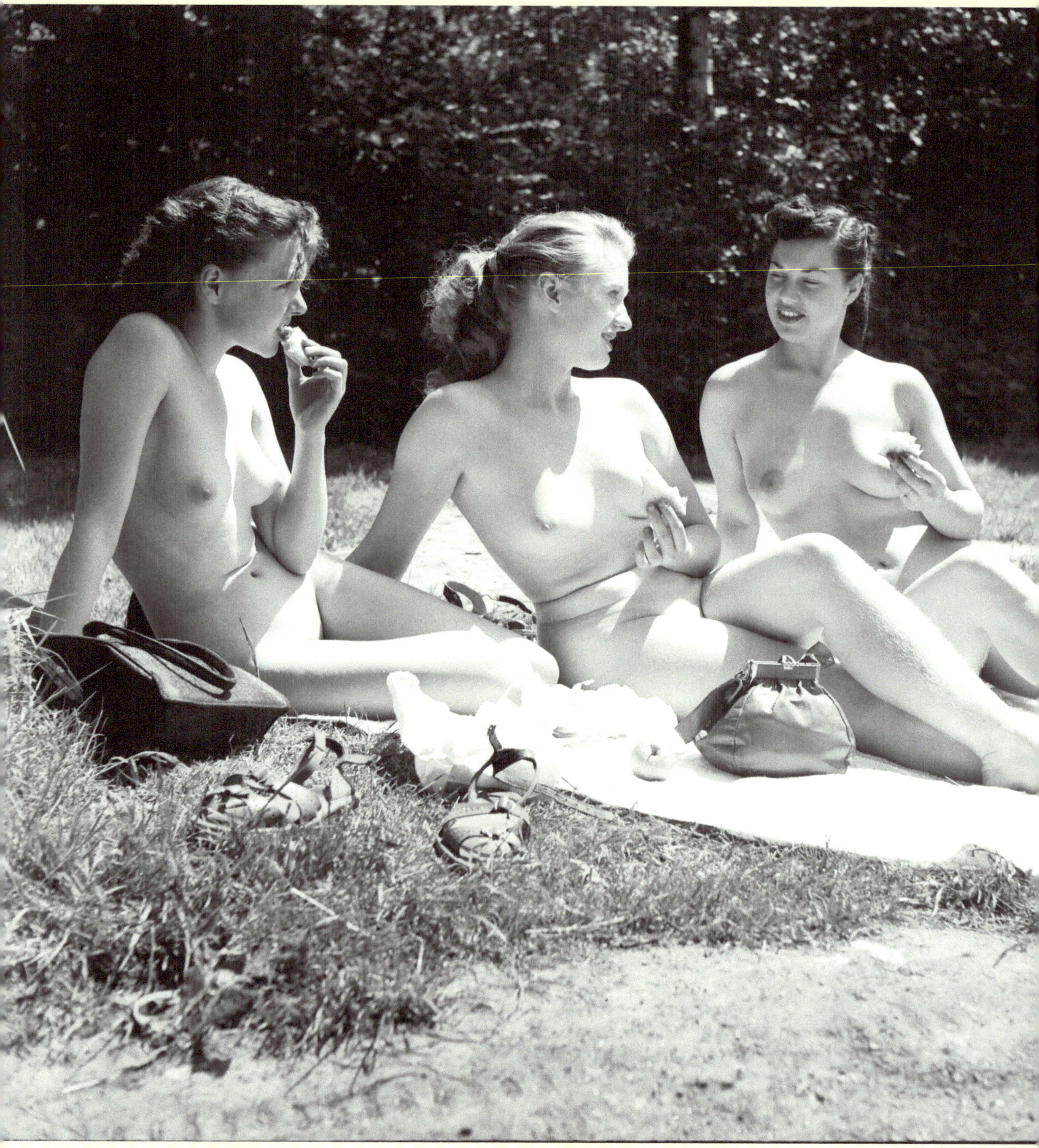

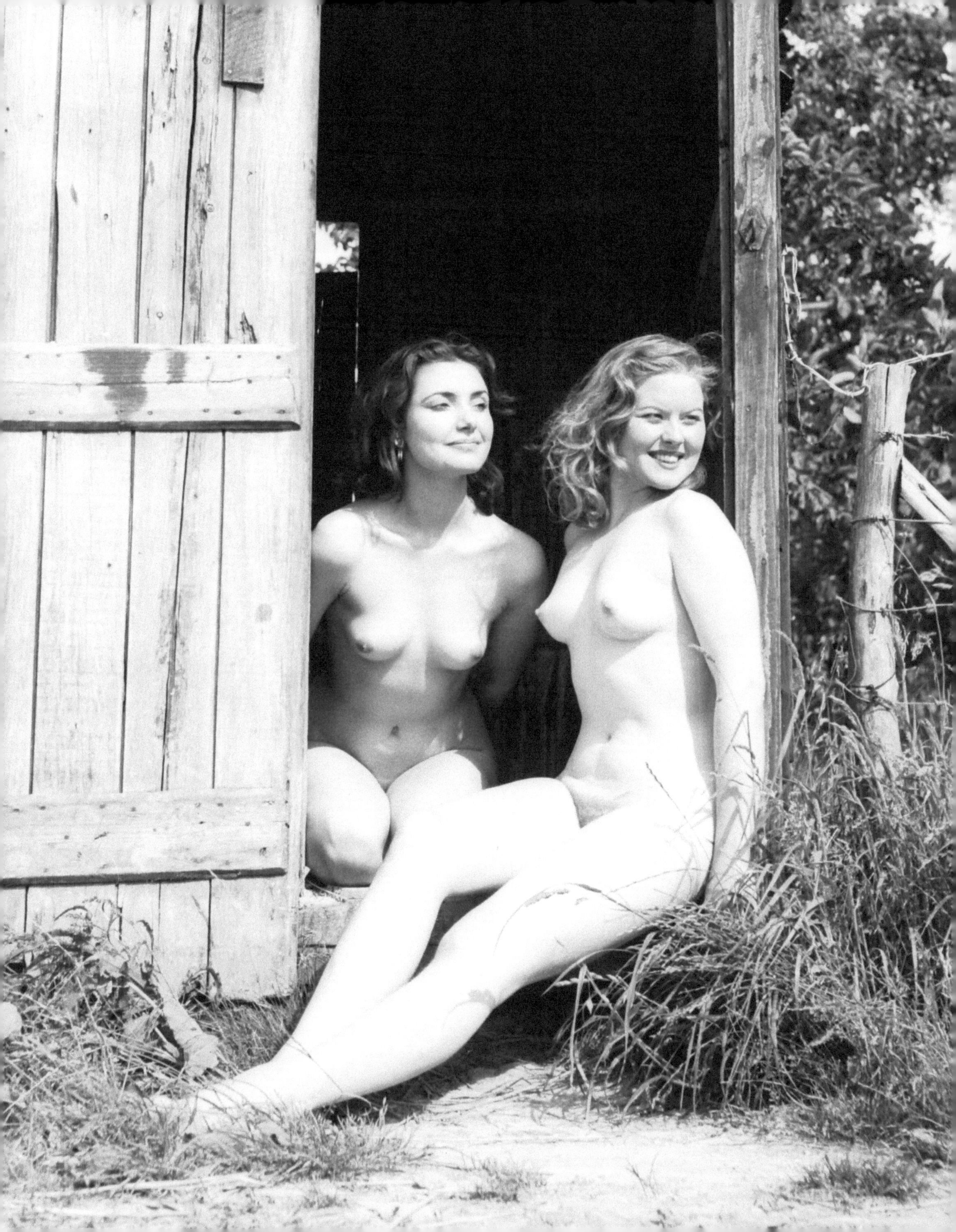

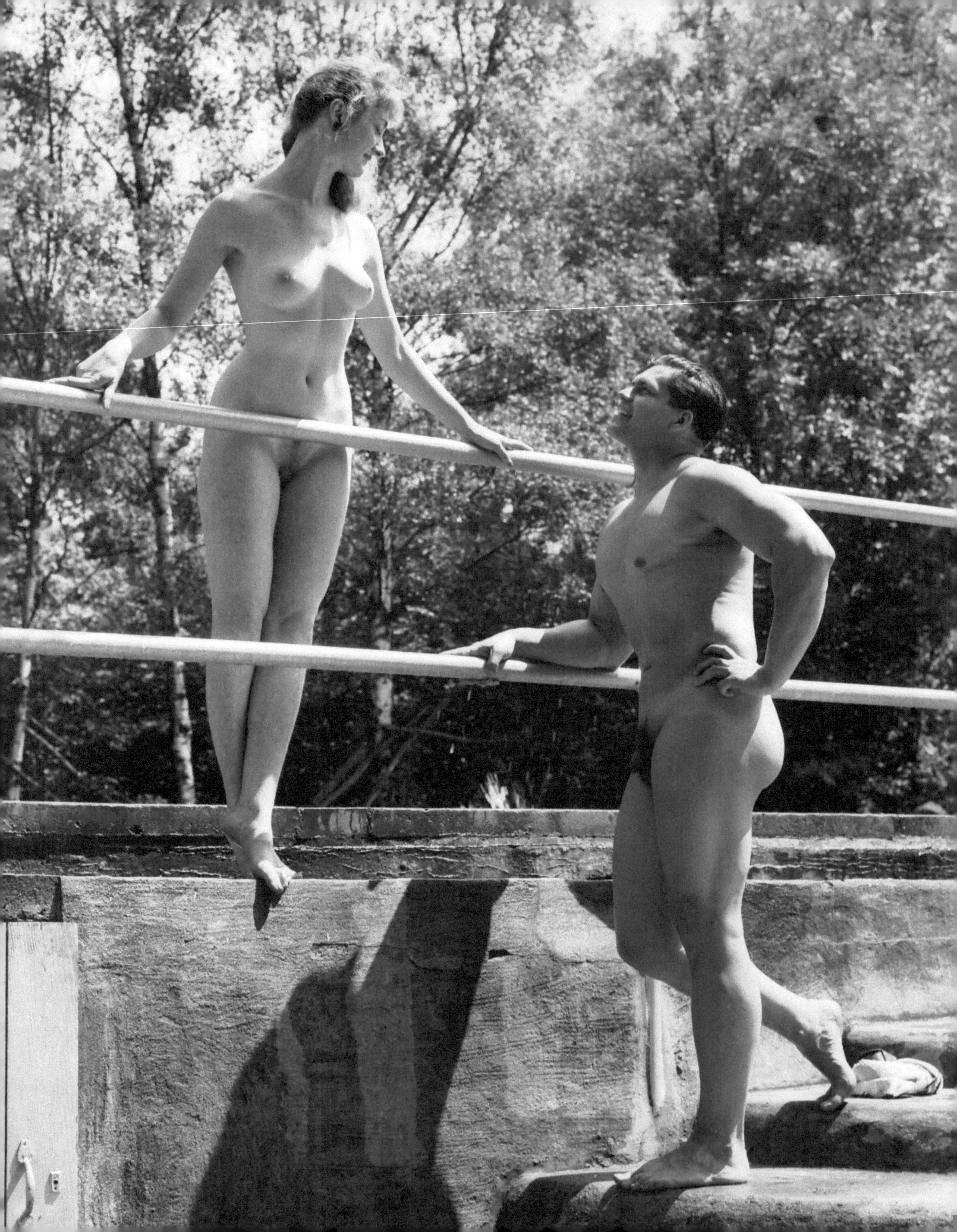

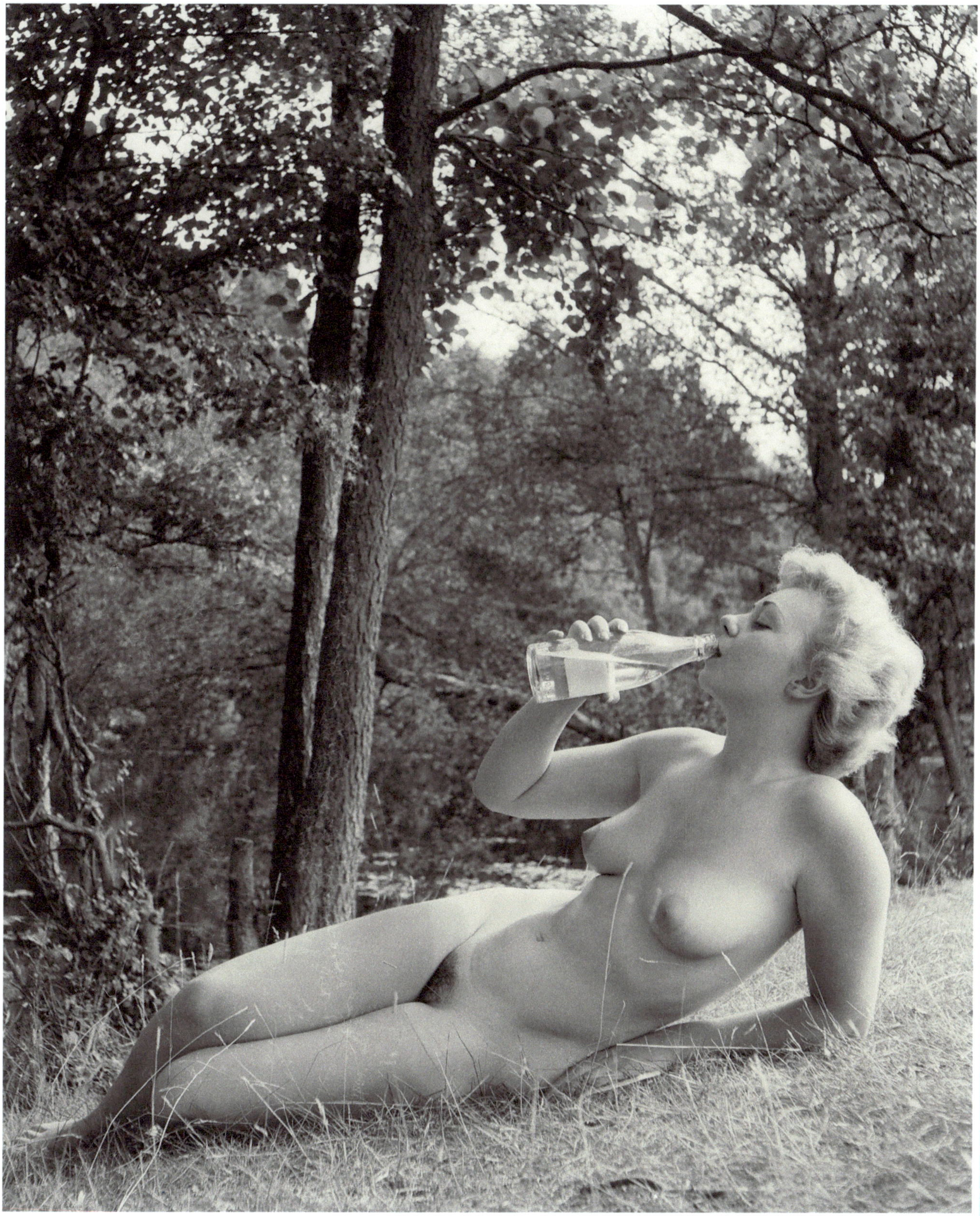

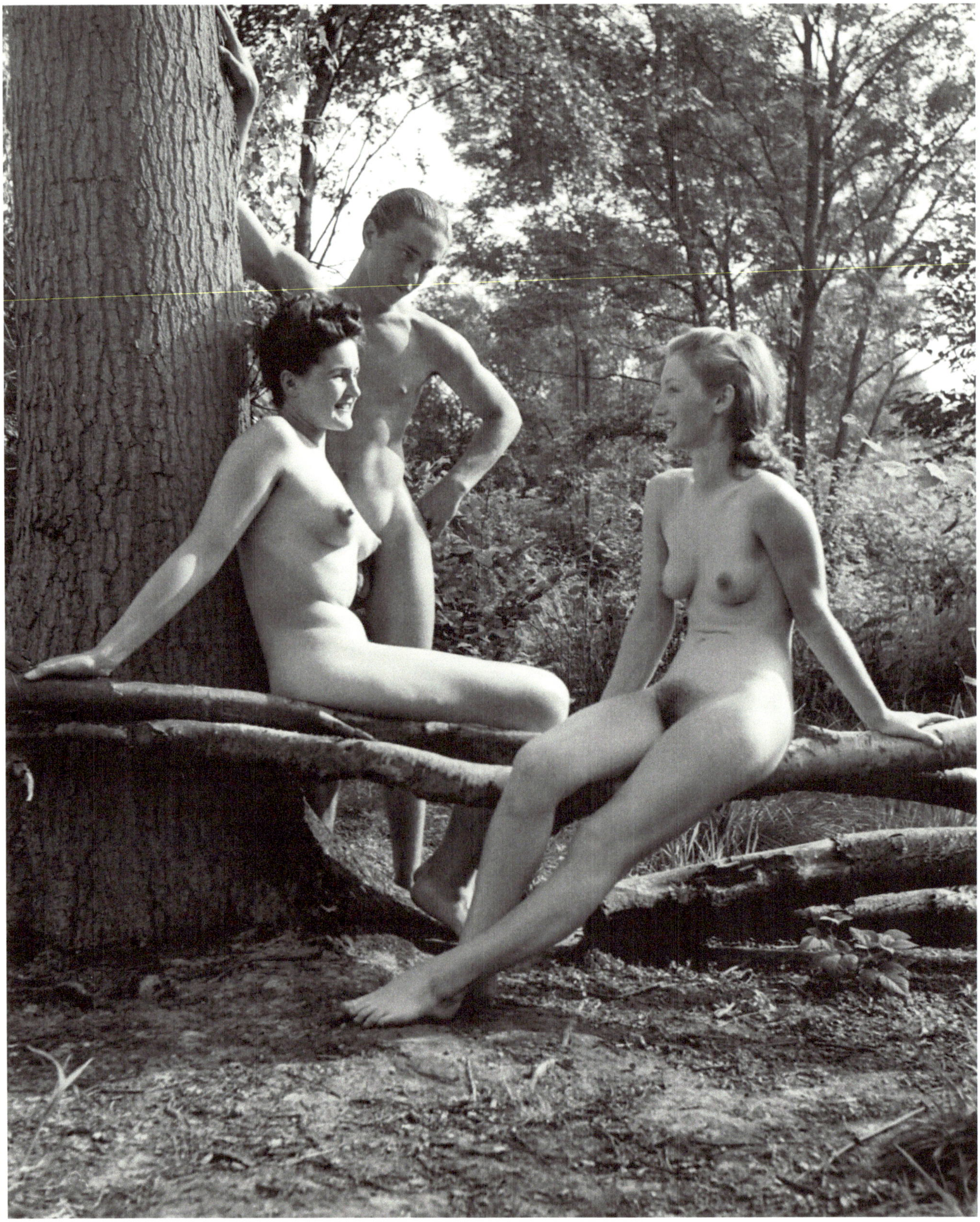

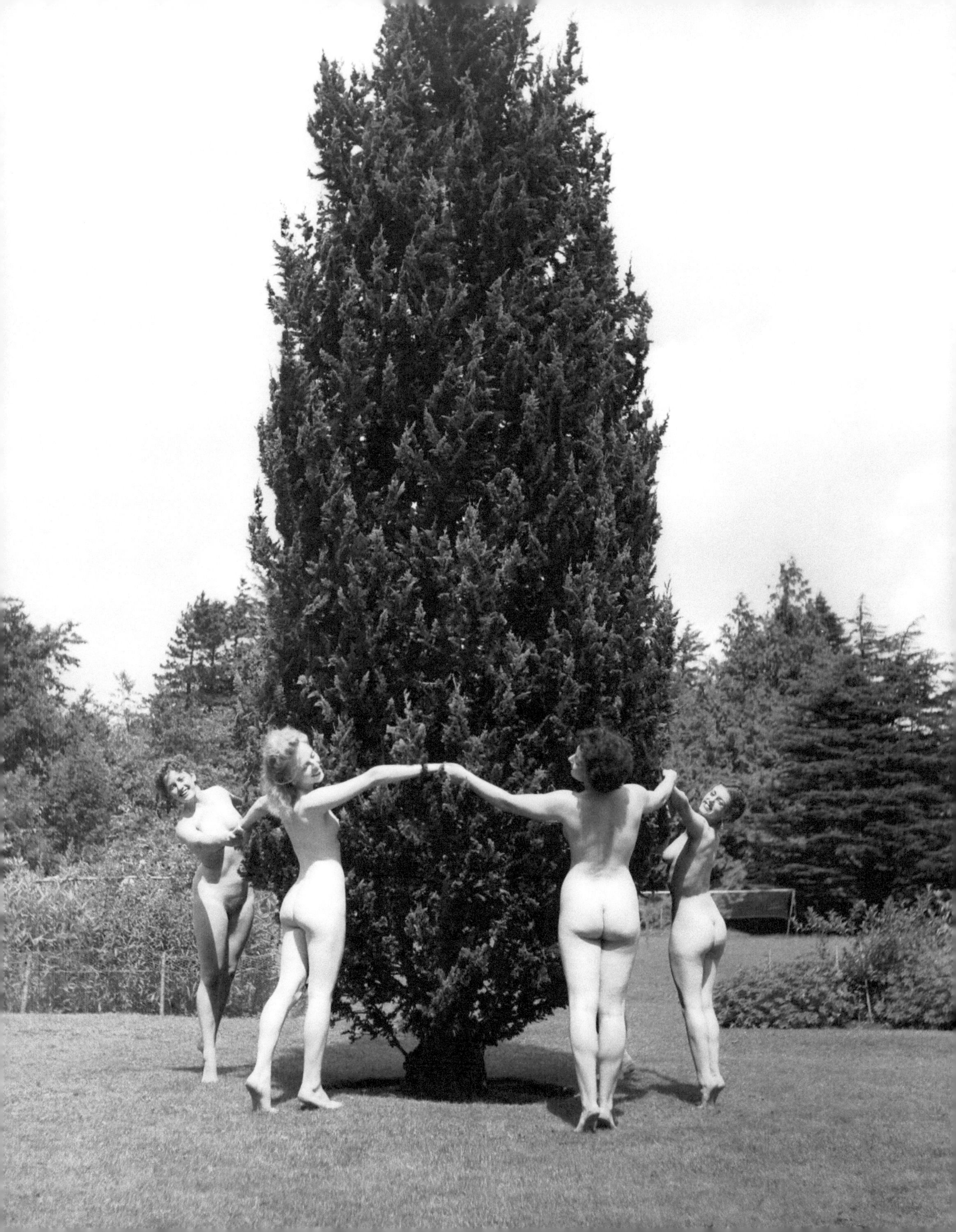

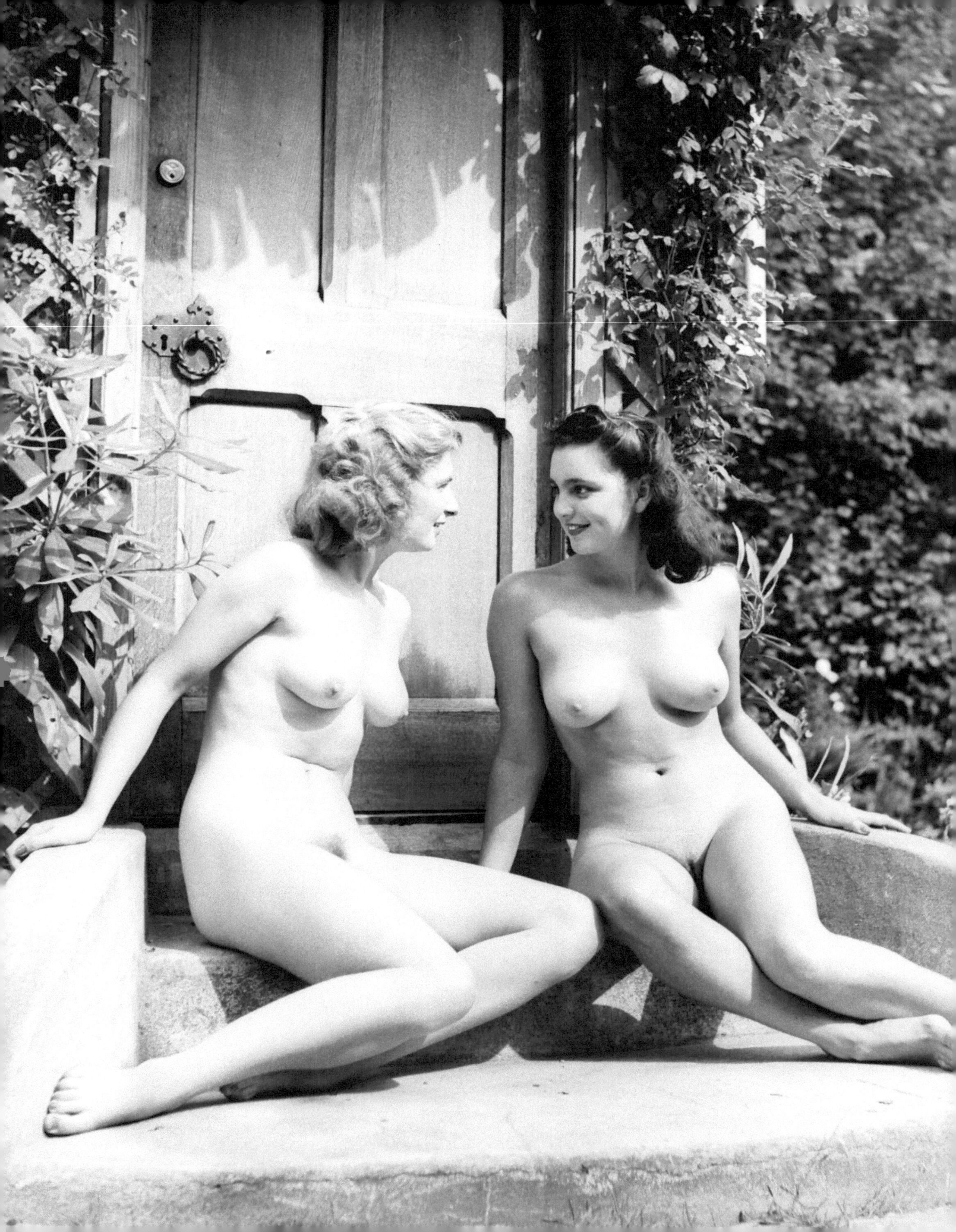

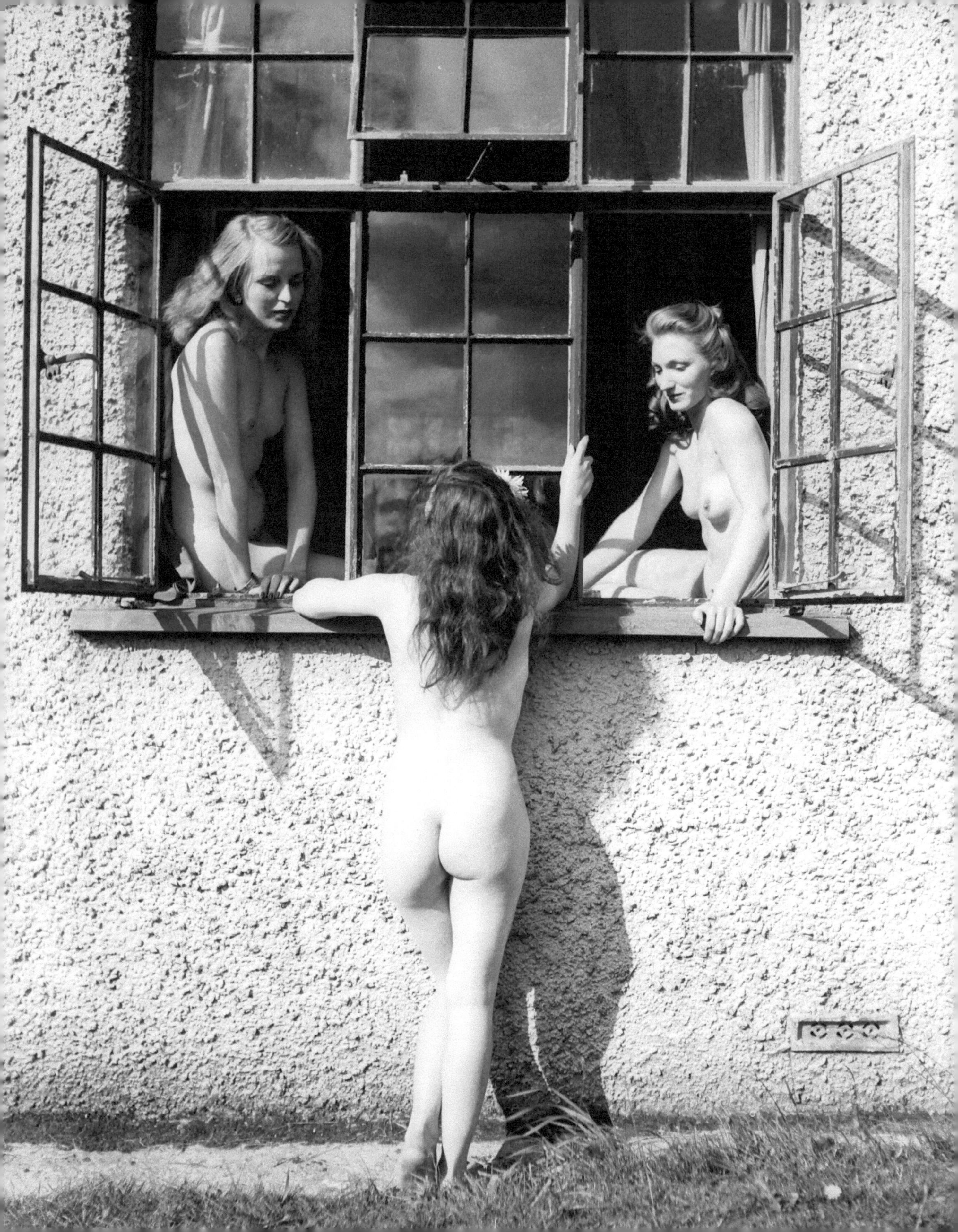

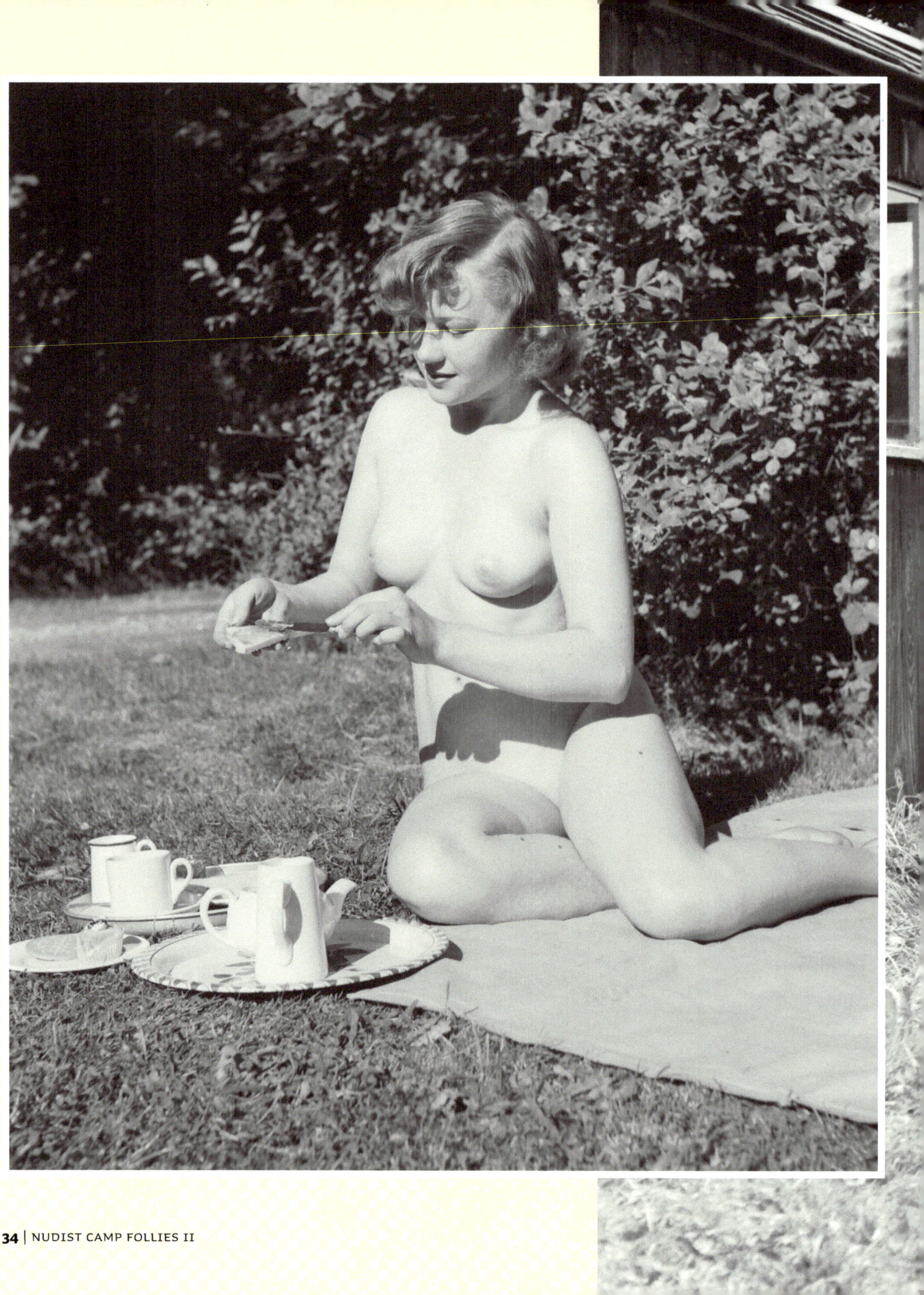

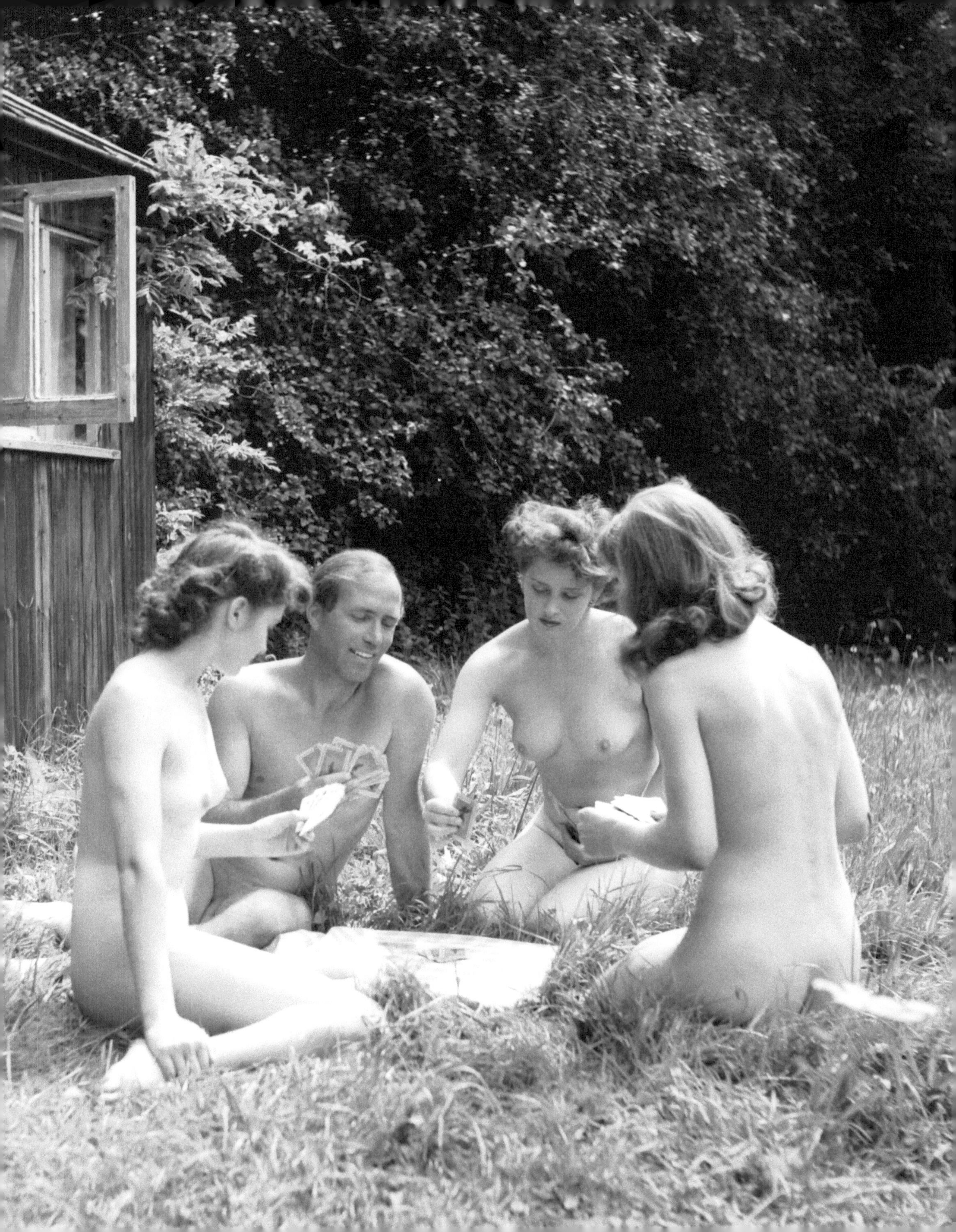

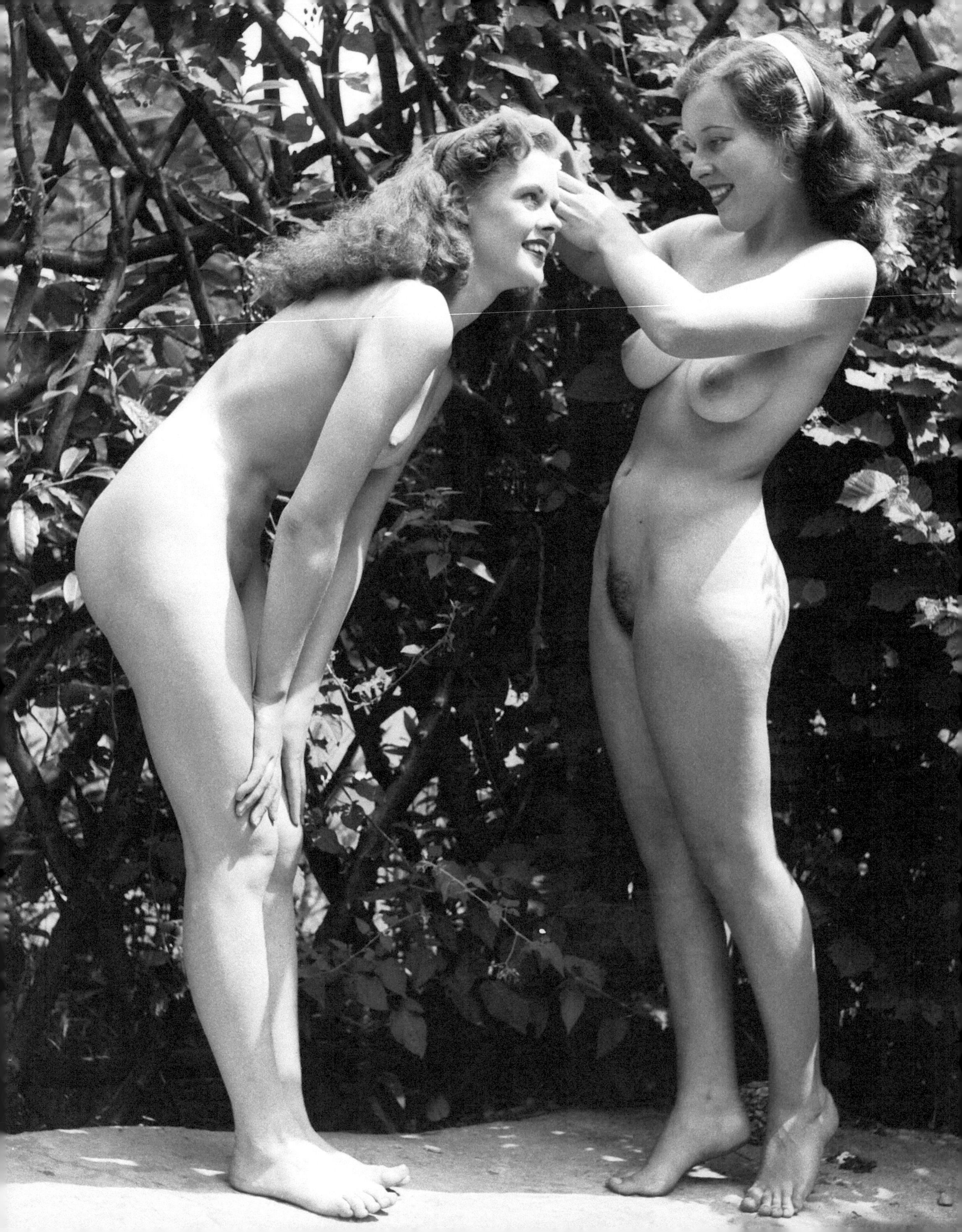

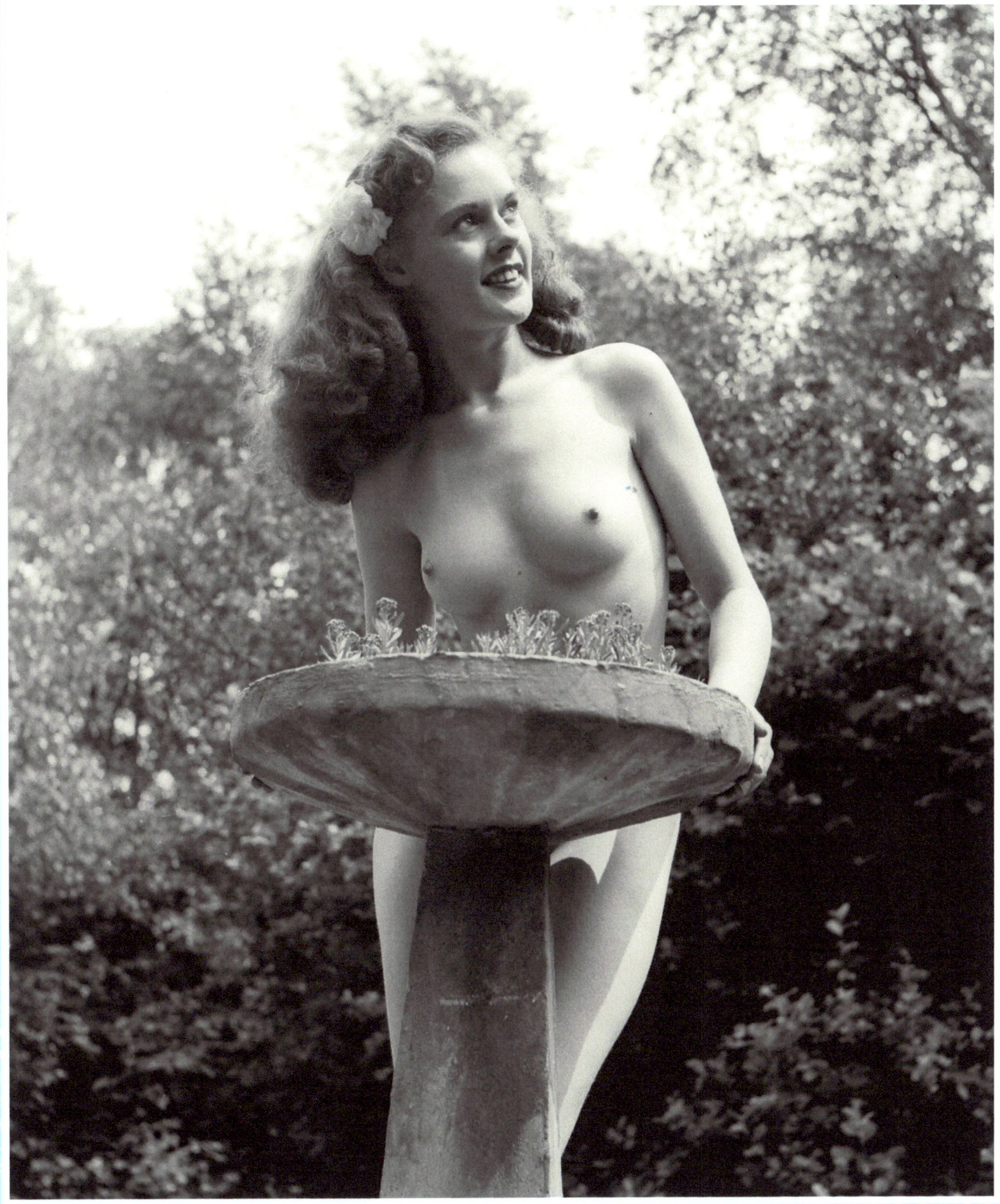

Above: Cover image of *Health and Efficiency*, December 1950.

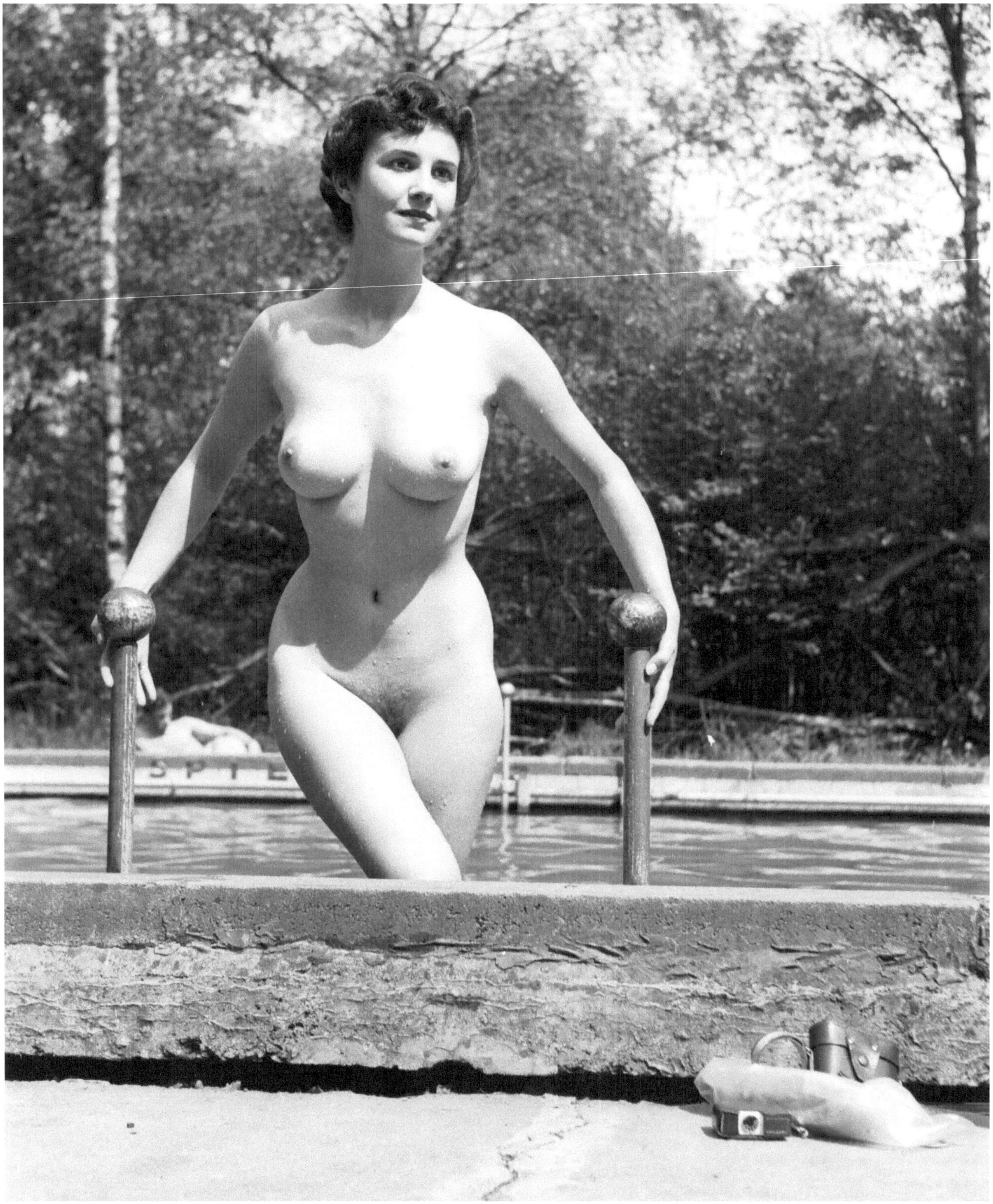

Above: Anita Smith. **Right:** Audrey Wayne and Anita Smith.

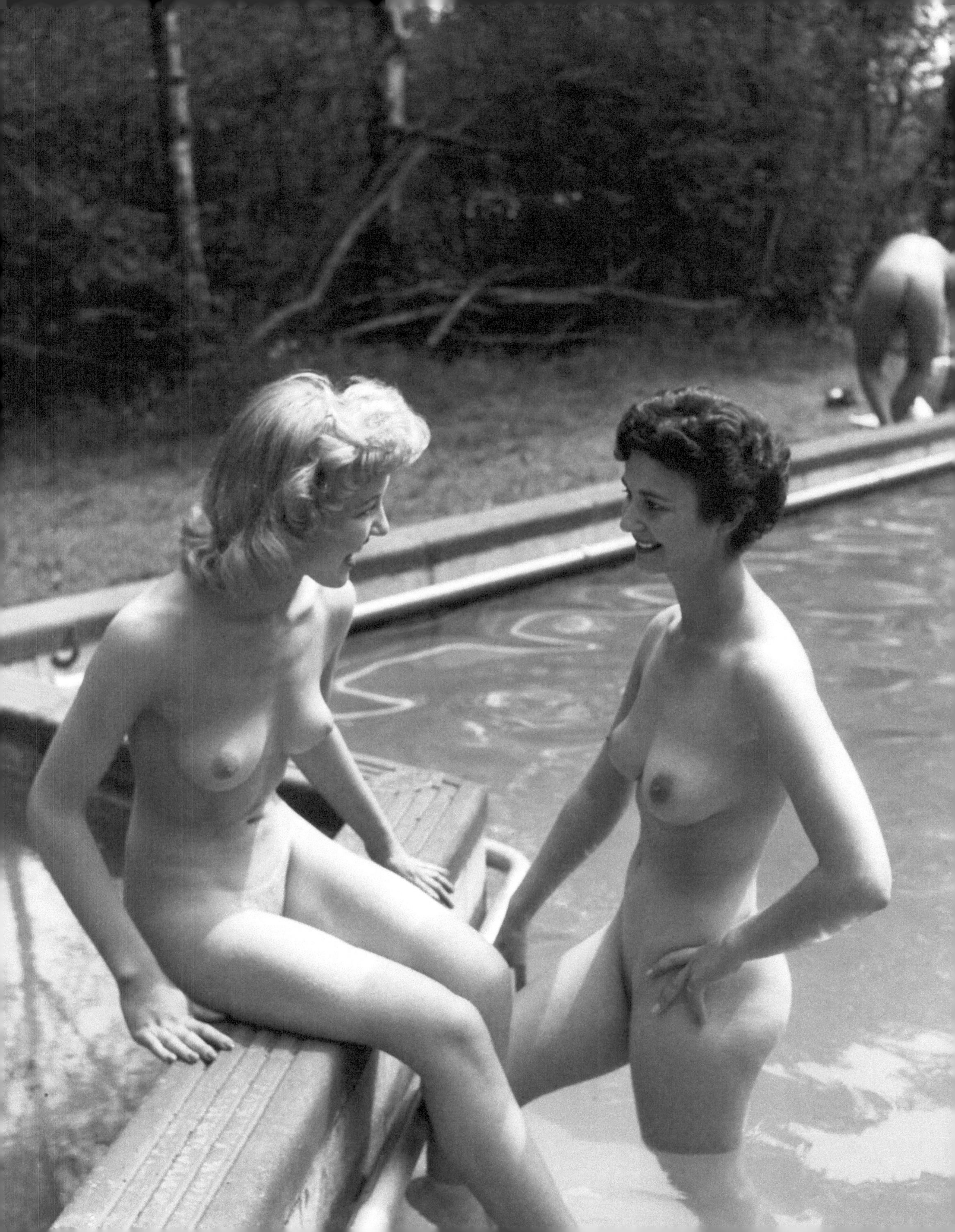

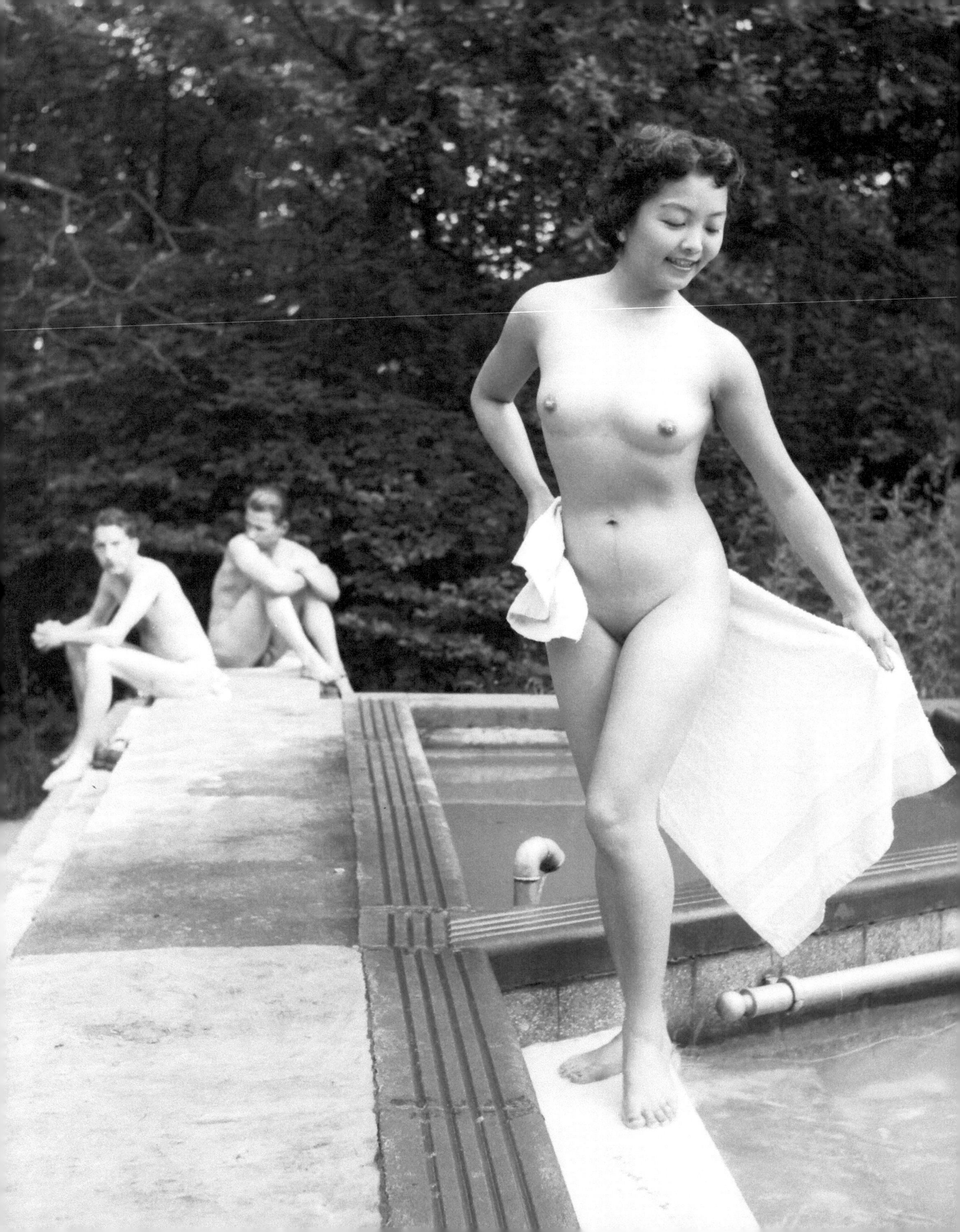

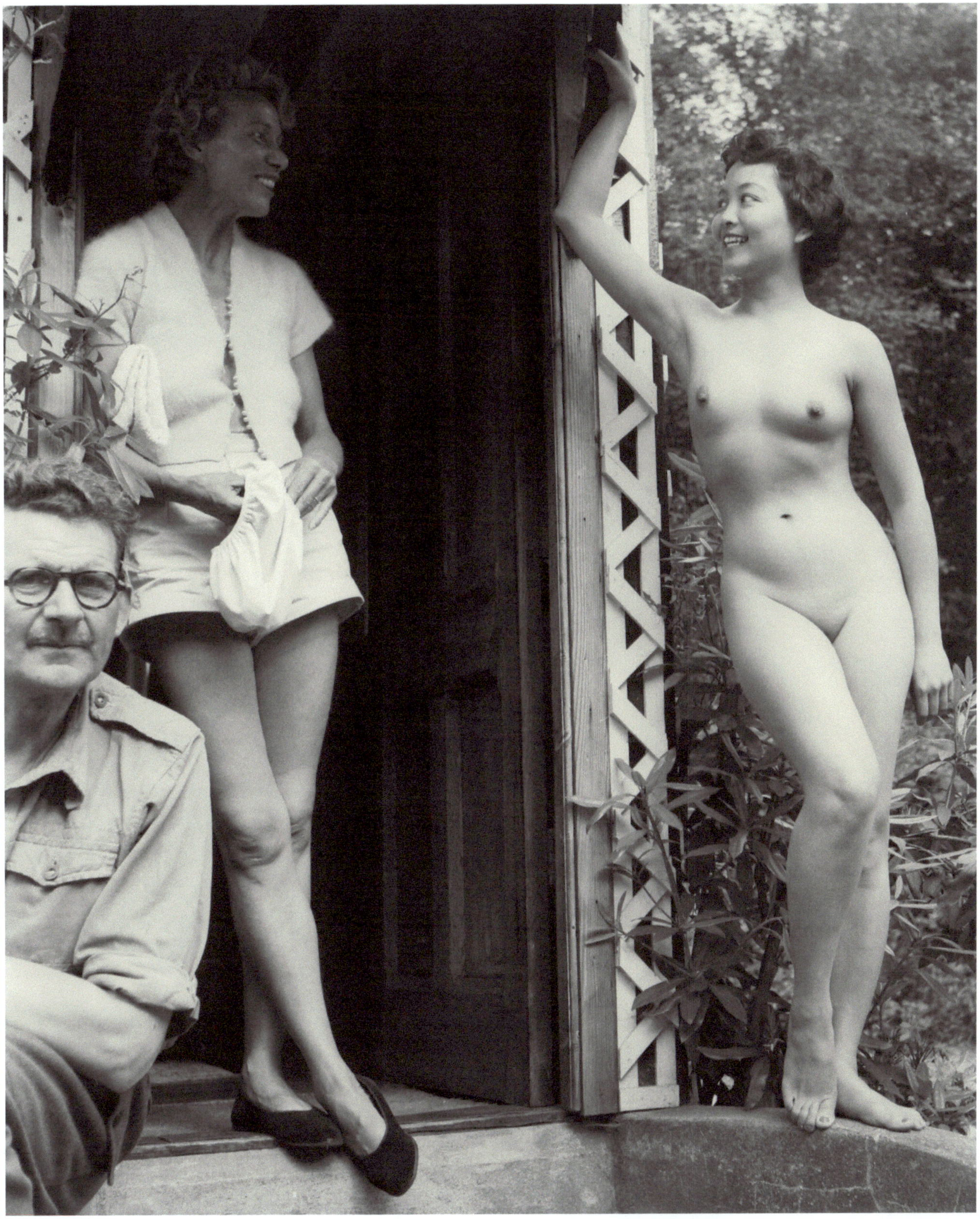

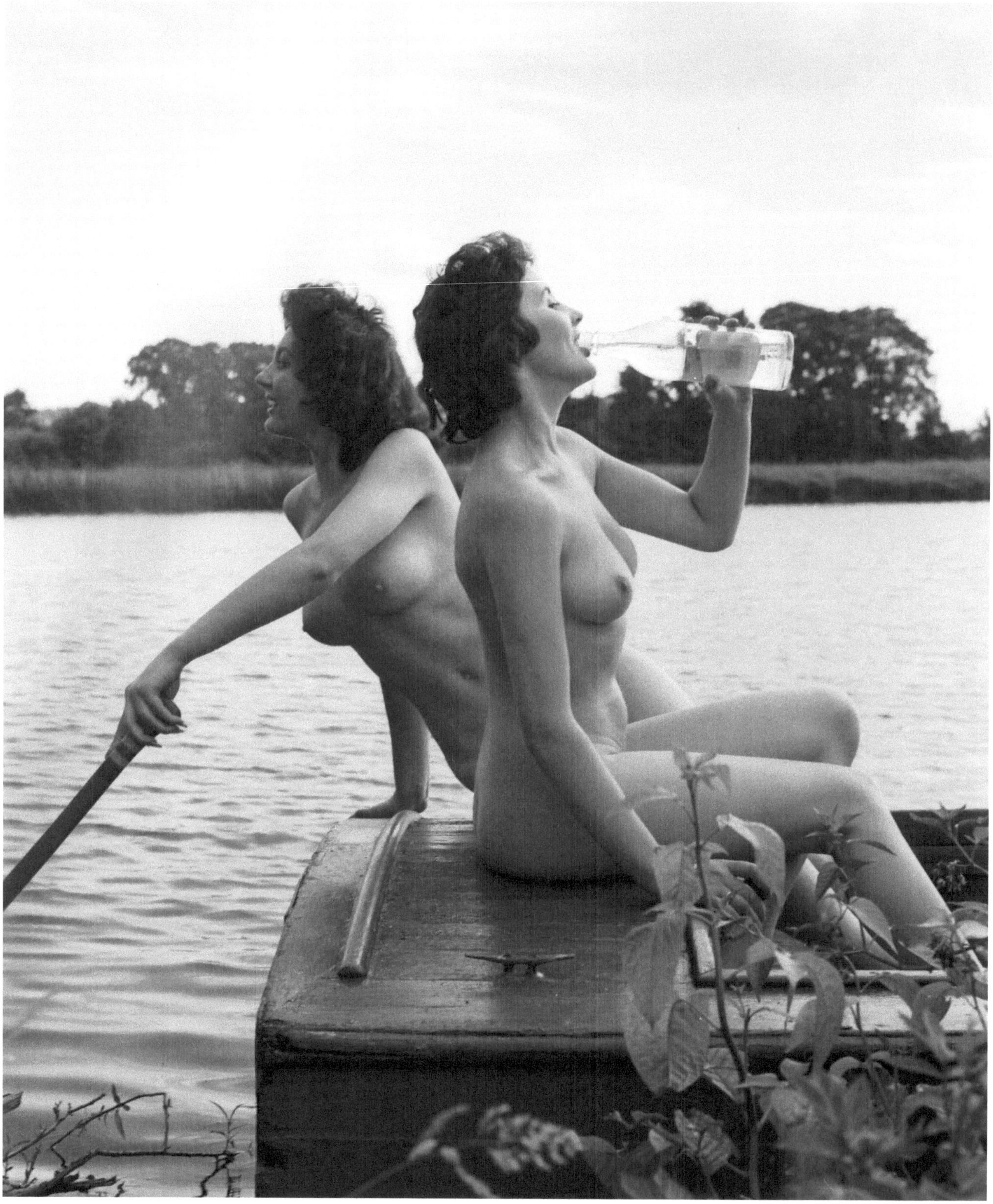

Above and right: The ever-popular Lee Sothern (left), with a friend.

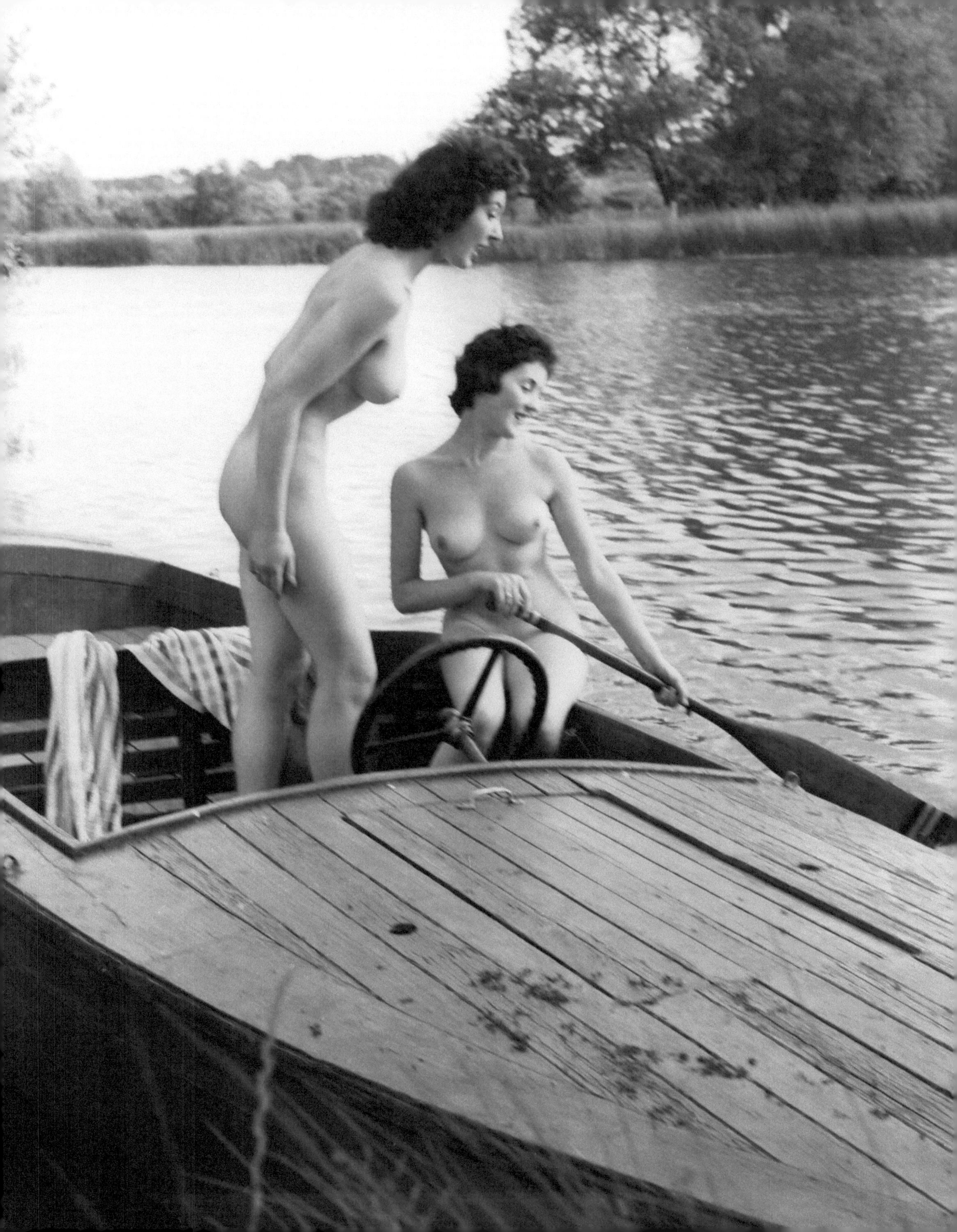

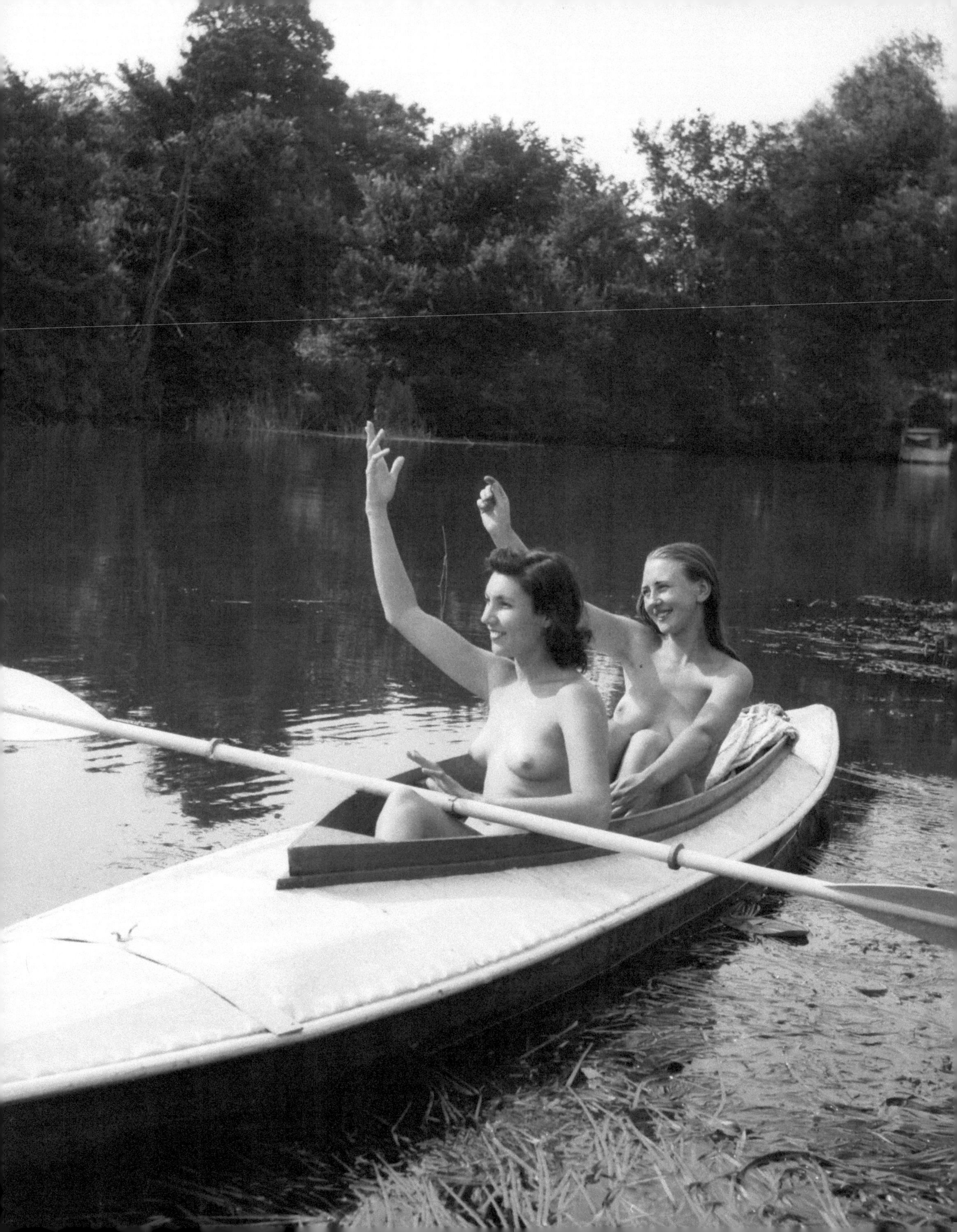

AVAILABLE TITLES FROM WOLFBAIT

Doing Rude Things
The history of the British sex film.

NEW! **Cinema au Naturel**
A history of nudist film.

Miniten: Rules of the Game
Invented in the 1930s, Miniten is a tennis-like game played by naturists.

Naked as Nature Intended
The epic tale of a nudist picture by Pamela Green, with photographs by Douglas "Dambuster" Webb, DFM.

The Naked Truth About Harrison Marks
The notorious biography by Franklyn Wood.

Past Masters of the Nude
An illustrated bibliography of nude photography books published in England from 1896 to 1960.

THE STEPHEN GLASS COLLECTION

Amazons of Yesteryear
A rare, action-packed collection of images of wrestling women of the 1940s and 1950s.

Beauty Off-Duty
Relaxed, everyday moments caught on camera.

Naked in the Menagerie
A playful look at Eve accompanied by her animal friends.

Nudist Camp Follies – volumes 1 and 2
An intimate look at the natural and free atmosphere in Sun Clubs.

Nymphs and Naiads
Beauty unadorned and outdoors.

NEW! **Poise and Pose**
A magnificent series of photographs of female beauty taken in the studio.

Order online at wolfbait.co.uk

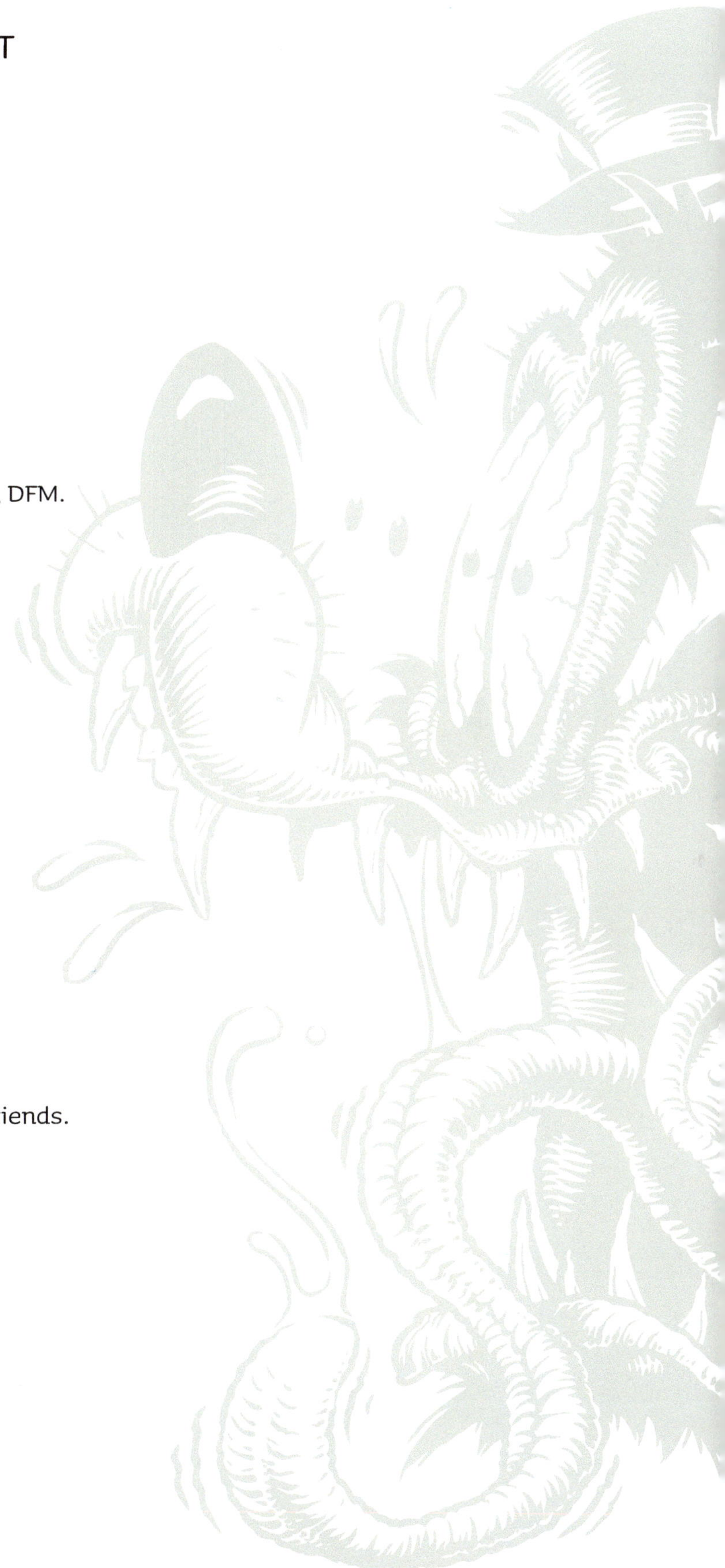

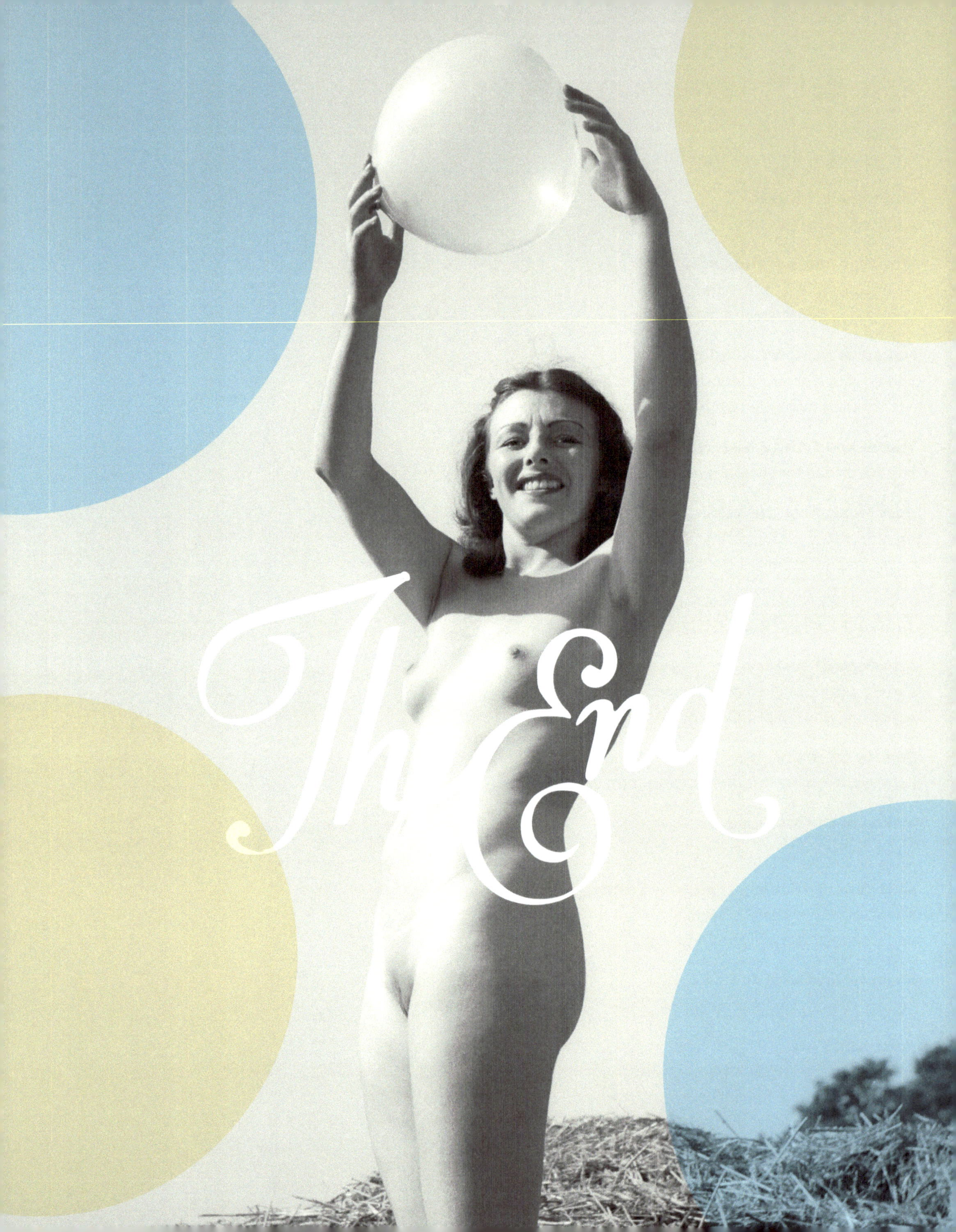
The End